OUTLIVE YOUR ENEMIES

Terry Sanford

Kroshka Books
New York

Cover Design: Maria Ester Hawrys

Art Director: Maria Ester Hawrys
Assistant Director: Elenor Kallberg
Graphics: Denise Dieterich and Kerri Pfister
Manuscript Coordinator: Roseann Pena
Book Editorial Production: Gavin Aghamore, Tammy Sauter
Circulation: Irene Kwartiroff and Annette Hellinger

Library of Congress Cataloging-in-Publication Data

Sanford, Terry, 1917-
  Outlive your enemies / by Terry Sanford
      p.   cm.
  Includes bibliographical references.
  ISBN 1-56072-289-4 (Hardcover: alk. paper0. -- ISBN 1-56072-278-9)
  (pbk.: alk. paper)
  1. Ages--Health and hygiene. 2. Longevity. 3. Aging. I. Title.
RA777.6.S26   1996
613'.0438--dc20   95-8061
                                                       CIP

Copyright © 1996 by Terry Sanford
                      Nova Science Publishers, Inc.
                      6080 Jericho Turnpike, Suite 207
                      Commack, New York 11725
                      Tele. 516-499-3103 Fax 516-499-3146
                      E Mail Novascil@aol.com

Printed in the United States of America

OUTLIVE YOUR ENEMIES

DEDICATION

The book is dedicated to my mother, Betsy (Elizabeth Terry Martin) Sanford, superb school teacher, who lived to her hundredth year, still driving her automobile (albeit without a renewed license the last year) and living alone in our old home, alert, optimistic, with replaced hip, but no walking cane (Heavens, no!).

CONTENTS

PREFACE: WHY THIS?

I got interested in aging because aging got interested in me. I also had a more professional interest. Duke University has been a leader in the study of aging, and I, as president, had the opportunity to lend support to this important research and dissemination, and to learn more about the subject. In the U.S. Senate, I asked to be on the Committee on Aging.

As you grow older--to grow older--you may need luck, but there is much that you can do. What you eat can improve your health and to some extent can deflect disease. You can beat to the draw illnesses by regular physical exams and self-examination. You can quit relatively few bad habits and prolong your life. It is never too late to maintain your strength and increase your muscle capacity, and the vitality of vital organs, by appropriate exercise.

There is good medical treatment for the diseases of the elderly, but our bright hope is the efficacy of preventive health care for the elderly, and the heartening aspect is that prevention can be mostly self-administered.

I needed to know more. There are many good books on aging, but no one that gave me exactly what I wanted. I began to "review the literature," reading what George Maddox of the Duke Center on Aging thoughtfully sent me from time to time. When I was in the U.S. Senate, the Library of Congress afforded me a look at all the appropriate literature I could handle. I had long before begun to compile the material in a personal notebook, so I could better understand how to stand up to age.

As this notebook process matured, it metamorphosed into a book, expressing what I wanted to know as I passed seventy-five while realizing more and more that I would have been better served had I discovered all this as I approached fifty. My memory chanced on the round table at the old Prince Charles Hotel in Fayetteville, North Carolina, where as a beginning lawyer I spent many delightful lunch hours with a dozen friends who gathered as their various schedules permitted, and where we solved the problems of the world, large and small. I would make my summary of aging a conversation between my old cronies grown older, now personally and directly concerned with the irreversible cadence of time.

I metaphysically gathered my old friends at breakfast, and let them chat. As I scrambled their personalities with others, they became real to me. I could no longer identify the individuals, nor can they. I got caught up in the fun of the exercise. This "study" became a hobby, itself a measure of preventive health therapy.

There is Henry Murphy. He is the more or less retired head of a family business, an electrical contracting firm founded by his grandfather. Henry felt compelled to come home to take over when his two uncles died in a short period. He had been teaching for a few years at the state university, and had earned his doctorate, ABD ("all but dissertation," as graduate students know). He never finished it. He hasn't lost some of the pedantry he acquired at the college lectern.

There is Joe Zaroom, second generation Lebanese. He played college baseball, returned from the War (i.e., World War II, "The War"), opened a bargain clothing store, ran it for some forty years, and two years ago had held what he called "A Gigantic Once-in-a-Lifetime Going Out of Business Sale." He sold almost everything, gave the rest to the Salvation Army and the key to the landlord, and walked away.

Joe had wanted to be a professional baseball player. He had followed the New York Yankees since he had been a little boy helping at his father's magazine stand., but had never quite got up the nerve to try professional ball. He wears a New York Yankees cap, indoors and out, which, Roddy Thomas suggests, is to cover his bald spot.

There is Rodney Thomas, relaxed, easy going, overweight, successful head of his local insurance agency. He says he is retired but he goes to his office every day.

There is Lear Jones, who did not go to college, earned a high school equivalency during the War, and became business manager of a large plumbing firm, active in the YMCA and other community civic work.

There is Victor Beane, the proud grandson of a slave, a U.S. Post Office employee since the War, a supervisor by the time he reached retirement age. He takes great pride in his heritage, in his accomplishments, and in his house and yard.

There is William McKeithan, Will Mack he is called, who dedicated himself to teaching, to the Boy Scouts, the Lions Club, his Sunday School class, his family, and most of all, his students. He had retired at the appointed time as the most beloved high school principal in the history of the county.

There are a few other participants, Violet, Gus, and John McCorn, but they will introduce themselves. The reader is invited to join us as the seventh old crony whenever we gather for breakfast.

Now, why would I, not a scientist, make bold to write on a scientific subject? That is a fair question. I thought it would be helpful for a layman to write to laymen on a complicated subject.

Others wondered why I did not write my impressions straight out, instead of gathering old friends to talk about it. That, too, is a fair question. Some of these scientific theories need to be disputed, are disputed, so it seemed useful to bring in contrary viewpoints and opinions. I hope the conversations will be helpful to the reader, and maybe entertaining. I hope that the reader as the seventh breakfast guest will feel free to get into the arguments and discussions.

This group of characters is more or less homogeneous, but a diverse group while better representing the populations of the aging, would not have gathered for easy conversation.

The breakfast buddies are not the biblical "poor, and the maimed, and the halt, and the blind," but they are concerned, as am

I, with the more painful, and sometimes shameful, conditions of the elderly.

It would have been neat, but not realistic, to have included women at the conversations, but the discussions and conclusions do relate equally to women. Many of the experts quoted are female. These cronies involve their wives in their home discussions, and observe the rules of better aging because the wives keep their feet to the fire.

In these conversations the cronies are focused on how they, ordinary older persons on their feet, can stay on their feet. They want to know how to conquer or at least encounter aging with dignity and self-esteem, in as good health as better habits might facilitate.

"It's luck," says Joe Zaroom. It is more than luck. That, too. These conversations are about what the experts say can lead to growing old and staying healthy--how we can enjoy life to the hilt to the end!

Acknowledgments

I am indebted to many people, especially Dr. George L. Maddox of Duke University's Department of Gerontology, who initially sparked my interest in aging as an academic subject, pointed me toward the right materials, and read my manuscript for any outrageous assumptions I might have slipped in.

I also thank Mary and Cecil Sanford, my brother and sister-in-law who are English scholars, Dr. Leslie Banner, author and Duke administrator, Shirley Cochrane, author and teacher, Judy Love, my Senate legislative assistant for the Select Committee on Aging, and William Green, public affairs vice president and teacher of journalism at Duke University, all of whom read the first manuscript and made constructive suggestions.

I thank Dr. James H. Billington and the Library of Congress for the red carpet help. Finally and especially, I am grateful to Marsha C. Vick, for her research and editorial assistance.

Chapter One

SIX CRONIES AND A VENTURE

*T*he door of the little brick bungalow swings open and out strides a husky man in blue pajama bottoms, hair tousled and somewhat dusty, not quite gray. He takes a few steps toward the newspaper lying at the edge of the drive, stops, stretches his arms outward and upward, takes a deep breath, stretches again as he slowly looks around at the sky and the yard, and says to himself, aloud, "Boy, a beautiful day!"

He takes another step or two, gingerly because he is barefooted, leans over to pick up the rolled newspaper, and says, again to himself and out loud, "These old bones are getting stiff. Got to get back to my exercise."

The sun, not yet in sight, is proclaiming its arrival, its white rays slithering through the trees. Paper in hand, Henry walks toward his three dwarf apple trees. He pauses, pulls down a branch of young leaves, observing little wormholes in several, and notes to himself, *Need to throw some mothballs around these roots.*

He turns and walks across the driveway to his shrubs. On the corner is an azalea bush, its dark green leaves highlighting tiny unopened buds. He stops, and somewhat ceremoniously, relieves his kidneys by spraying the azalea. *Best medical test in the world. When it dies I'll go to a doctor.* This is Henry Murphy.

He goes in and closes the door, and almost an hour has passed when Henry next comes out, dressed in gray suit and a flowered tie, freshly shaved, hair neatly combed. He walks down his driveway and along the edge of the street, whistling a jaunty little tune, musing to himself, *Springtime--look at the buds--soon fishing and baseball and strawberry shortcake--and flowers--and peaches.*

At Freedom Street, he steps to the sidewalk and consciously walks a little more briskly, straightens his shoulders, brushes his hair with his hand, feels the knot of his tie and finds it in place, runs his finger on his fly and finds it closed, deliberately moves his lips to a smile, and waves to the driver of the first car to pass. *They know I like to walk.*

Six blocks to go. The sun is just poking its red shoulder over the Millers' two-story furniture store. Now Henry reaches Main Street, turns and quickens his pace. He glances at his reflection in the window of the Western Auto Store, sucks in a deep breath, draws in his stomach, *Good looking feller, isn't he?* Halfway down the block is the U.S. Grill, its name painted on its two storefront glass windows, a waving Old Glory painted between a gold "U" and "S," with "GRILL" below, and still lower in smaller black print, "and restaurant."

Henry pushes on the door latch, the brass trigger shiny where countless thumbs had touched it, black elsewhere from weathering. Inside he glances to the back of the restaurant and then to his left, where an amiable gray-haired man with a neatly trimmed, snow-white mustache stands behind a cash register set atop a glass showcase filled with candy bars, boxes of cigars, and indigestion tablets.

"Morning, Gus," Henry beams.

Gus, smiling broadly, responds, "Wonderful day, Mr. Murphy."

Gus has on a gray cotton jacket, a spotless white shirt, and a little black bow tie so meticulously tied that it obviously is the snap-on variety. On a cabinet behind Gus is an adding machine, the old model with a summit roll of paper, along with piles of invoices and bills, scattered and stacked.

Henry Murphy makes for the rear of the cafe, along a counter facing circular stools bolted to the floor. The floor is of little white and black octagonal tiles set in a geometric pattern. To his right are tables for four, and high-backed booths along the wall. A lone man sits at the first table, and a woman and man occupy one of the booths, eating industriously and silently. At the back, next to the kitchen door, is a family table surrounded by eight chairs, wicker-bottomed, walnut-stained.

It is to this table that Henry is proceeding so intently. On the near side of the table sit two men; at the far end next to the booths sits another. They are sipping coffee from heavy white cups with a blue band around the top. There are two aluminum napkin holders guarded by salt and pepper shakers, a cluster of bottles--catsup, steak sauce, and hot sauce--a sugar bowl, and no tablecloth. A waxed pint milk carton sits in the middle of the table.

By this time Henry's broad grin turns into an open-mouthed smile.

"Morning!"

"Hi, Henry, you're late," says the man in the corner.

"Morning, " chime the other two.

"Morning Roddy. Joe Boy. I'm ahead of schedule," says Henry, still smiling. "Trouble with you, Lear, is you can't sleep. Guilty conscience."

Lear Jones nods agreement. "Sure is a pretty day. Done weeded my strawberries this morning." His tone is relaxed, languid. Harsh wrinkles splay from the edges of his droopy eyes. His face, gray to pink, is weathered like fine leather, his upper lip creased like a peeled tangerine. His graying hair, sparse against his tanned skull, looks as if it had not and could not be combed. Lear's mouth is turned more to a grin of amusement than a smile.

Henry sits down and takes a drink from a glass of water already placed there. A young woman in a waitress's white smock brings him a cup of coffee. "Good morning, Mr. Murphy."

"Good morning, Violet. That's what I need!"

Henry squares his chair around so he can see his three companions. "Time to prune the roses. The forsythia are beginning to bloom."

"I'm going to let my bushes fend for themselves this year," says a bear of a man sitting across from Henry. "I was looking yesterday and figured everything had a head start on the grass and weeds. I'm going to sit around and watch the flowers and the weeds race. Helen is betting on the weeds. I'm betting on the flowers."

"O.K., Roddy, it'll give me an excuse to bring roses to your wife," says Henry. "How is Helen?"

"'Bout the same, thanks for asking. She's doing what the doctor tells her."

Roddy--Rodney Thomas--wears a brown sweater and a shirt with an unbuttoned collar. His face is Scot, ruddy with brown splotches, eyes bright blue, the tone of his voice puckish, his chubbiness begins at his neck and ripples downward and outward. His tweed jacket hangs on his chair.

"None of you've got it made like me and Emma," says the little man sitting next to Roddy. "The condominium people do all the work. Chop all the weeds. Water the flowers. Rake the leaves." He has a small head dominated by sparkling, darting black eyes. He is wearing a New York Yankees baseball cap. His verbal tone is abrupt, final, the demeanor of a baseball umpire.

"But you don't get to pick the roses, Joe Boy," says Lear.

This is Joe Zaroom. "I can smell them. I'll settle for that."

Two other men are coming from the front of the restaurant.

"We're ready to order, Violet," calls Rodney. "The Hardy Boys are here."

"Hope you didn't wait for us," says one of the men. "Vic's alarm clock is broken--so he says." The speaker is gaunt, over six feet tall, his eyes sunken, his beard outline showing through his yellowed skin, but his facial expression is open, beckoning, friendly. This is William McKeithan--called Will Mack. He is a retired school teacher and principal.

"Not so," says Victor. "It is just that Will Mack is a slow driver. He wants to look at all the girl joggers." Victor Beane is plump, wearing a green woolen sport shirt, and is shiny bald except for a gray fringe over each ear extending down to scraggly sideburns. He wears a hearing aid tucked in his left ear.

Violet arrives at the table, her order book in hand.

"I'll take the usual," Henry nods to Violet. "So will I," says Lear.

"I'll have prunes and a bowl of oatmeal," says the plump one with the hearing aid.

"Prunes!" Lear's droopy eyelids pop wide open. "Good God, Victor, you'll be turning in to the hospital next."

Vic Beane smiles. "Prunes, Violet."

"Yes, Mr. Beane." She looks at the gaunt one. "What's for you, Mr. MacKeithen?"

Will Mack's sunken eyes are warm and bright, and his voice is soft and sunny. "Well, I was going to have prunes but I don't want the flap that comes with them. I'll take eggs, potatoes, sausage, and a side dish of cholesterol."

"I can handle that." Violet completes her notations and goes to the kitchen.

"Zaroom, you getting the Little League going this year?" Will Mack asks the little man with the Yankee's cap.

"Well, Will, we don't mess with that 'til closer to the end of school. But I'll be in there. Wouldn't miss it. You know Clyde Miller's boy Tim is the leading hitter at State? Batting four-twenty. I'm the one first taught him to hold a bat. His voice has a slight tone of arrogance, the baseball umpire. Mighty good players have come out of that program. The Zimmerman boy, captain of the high school team this year. He could make the pros. I don't recommend the pros. Too chancy. I recommend college. We've got this fellow that's come here with the Budweiser people who's going to coach one of my teams. I went out there to see him yesterday, and Herman will let him off. Played in the semi's three years. Knows his stuff."

"Now hold on there, Joe Boy," drawls Lear. "You about to get into the World Series and we ain't finished basketball yet."

"Well, it's about finished! Indiana got blown out last night."

"You don't see that too often."

"I thought they'd make it to the finals."

"Lotta luck when you get that far," says Joe of the Yankee's cap. "There's no predicting."

Rodney Thomas squirms. "Yes, there is luck in everything. You fellows didn't know him as well as I did. John Baratelli died yesterday. Fifty-two years old. Picture of health two weeks ago--work to do--great family, beautiful kids, talented wife, married 30 years. Children all out of college. Just getting where he could enjoy life. Worked hard, pinched pennies, finally made it. Then, zap! Dead. Heart attack. No warning. Zap! Funeral tomorrow afternoon. There ain't no justice."

"Well," says Will Mack, "Sorry to hear that. I know him. Taught his children. But I'd say there's justice on earth. We just don't understand how to measure it, how to recognize it, but we have to believe all works out for the best, somehow."

"No, there ain't no justice!," says Roddy. "Why do so many bright young people die, and so many old goats live forever?"

"Don't knock it. Look at the old goats around this table."

"I'd say we're all pretty lucky old goats. Here we are. Walking. Made it through depression and war. Ups and downs. Finally up-- somewhat. We are entitled to be cantankerous old goats."

"What do you suppose makes some people last and some people get called in early?," asks Victor. "I look at the kids I went to high school with. Dead! Most of them. Or blind, or crippled, or living--existing--in a rest home.

"Luck," says Joe Zaroom. "Nothing you can do about it. Luck. It takes luck to reach old age. And we ain't there yet. I quit the store just in time."

"I remember a man in my neighborhood when I was a boy." It is Rodney Thomas, in his puckish tone. "He was going to live to be a hundred. Told everybody he was. Real health nut. Took ten kinds of vitamins. Went out running every morning, long before that became a craze. Did pushups and calisthenics. Would get up from a party to go home when his bedtime came. Eight hours sleep. Wouldn't take a drink and long since quit smoking. Wouldn't eat greasy foods. Even at the church picnic he would pull all that good crisp skin off of fried chicken. Went to church regularly. What happened to him? Where did it get him?

"Out running one rainy morning, slipped in the mud on the shoulder of the road, slid under a log truck. Dead at fifty!"

"Damn!," says Lear. "But if he hadn't been running he might have ended up with a stroke and a cane."

"Give me the cane," says Joe.

"I was always sorry he didn't make it," says Roddy. "I sorta thought I wanted to follow his example, do things that would let you live to be old, really old, to see what was going on. I reckon I lost interest in trying when he got killed."

"Don't worry, Roddy," Will Mack says, "you can still live to be a hundred. Lots of people do. It is a matter of what you eat and how you work and how you take care of yourself. My father died with a heart attack when he was forty. I've already lived over fifty percent longer than he did, over twice as long as an adult. That's why I don't smoke. Doctor made me quit thirty years ago. That's why I don't work very hard. My daddy worked twelve hours a day, six days a week, and I'm still here and haven't ever been in a hospital bed. And I want to be here a long time more."

"Wait a minute," says Henry, laughing. "Hard work won't kill you. I heard the mayor at your testimonial say you worked sixteen hours a day at Grainger High for thirty years."

"That wasn't work."

"Well, fellers," says Victor Beane, "it's a somewhat morbid thought, but how many of us will be here next year? Five years?"

"Hell, this table will be worn out before we are," says Lear.

"Or old Gus will be bankrupt," says Roddy.

"Or they'll tear down the place for urban redevelopment."

"Yes," Will Mack says. "And they'll have found the cure for cancer, and we will have found a way to settle differences without going to war, and we will have eliminated hunger in the world. I'd like to be here to see all that. It would be great to be alive and alert and healthy for the next twenty-five or thirty years. But, sad to say, old friends, we are not likely to make it."

"Why not?" Victor asks. "You remember reading a book review in the paper some time ago about a village somewhere in Afghanistan or the Ukraine, where everybody lived to be more than a hundred? Everybody in this country expects to live to be sixty-five and then that's the end. The law says so. Social Security says so. You are old when you get to be sixty-five. They threw me out of the Post Office. Can't work. Get ready to die. In Afghanistan those birds live so far back in the hills they don't know any better. They don't know you are supposed to die when you are sixty-five. They think the thing to do is to work and live forever. Pure ignorance keeps them living. You know my grandfather was a slave and I remember him well. He lived to be a hundred and one. Didn't know he shouldn't. Didn't have Social Security."

Lear Jones is hunched, listening intently. He pushes his egg-stained plate away, leans forward, his long forefinger, browned and rough, tapping on the table. "Let me tell you something. By God I intend to live at least thirty more years, maybe forty." He slowly draws a circle on the table with his finger, and then quickly fills it with a check mark. "If you can live one decade you can live an-other." And he slowly draws another circle, and quickly puts a check in it. "You can live longer than you think." And he slowly draws another circle and puts a check in it. "Let me tell you some-thing. I resent the hell out of being retired. I'm the best man they had. I know more than anybody there. I wasn't ready to quit, and don't intend to die." And he draws very slowly another larger circle and fills it quickly with three crosses. "And the whole Ridenhour crowd down there can kiss my ass. I'll be here when they're all gone."

Nobody speaks. Tears well in his eyes.

Quickly Rodney Thomas claps the table and speaks up. "You are right, Lear, old buddy, you are right. By golly, I'm with you. Reminds me of a story. Seems there was this church revival and the preacher was talking about loving your enemies, forgiving trans-gressions, and brotherly love. He swelled with his subject, and he called on the congregation for testimony. 'Tell me,' he called out, 'Is there a soul among this Christian congregation who can honestly say that he has not a single enemy in the world?' No hand moved. 'Tell me,' the preacher cried again, 'Is there not someone here who doesn't have a single enemy?'

"A stooped old man who had his palm cupped to his ear, slowly raised his hand. 'Wonderful, wonderful, wonderful! Brother Peterson, tell this congregation how you have reached your ripe old age without a single enemy.'

"The old man, sitting in the third pew from the front, slowly creaked to a standing position and turned around and unhurriedly surveyed the whole congregation. Then he croaked, as loudly as he could, 'I outlived the sons of bitches!' "

Everybody laughs, especially Lear. "Tell you what we ought to do," said Joe Zaroom, "Let's get that book and find out what caused them Afghanies to live so long. Where can we get that book?"

"Why you dodo," Henry Murphy laughs, "from the library, that's where they keep books. In libraries."

"Tell you what," says Victor Beane, pointing to Henry, "Let's commission the professor to find the book and review it for us. He knows all about libraries and lecturing and all that stuff. Even writes book reviews for the newspaper."

"Great idea."

"Yeah, Henry, get the book and give us the secrets."

Henry smiles. "That's not a bad project, but let me tell you turkeys something. I never could put up with dull students. I'll get the book and tell you what's in it, if you'll pay attention. For that matter, I'll do it anyhow. I'll learn something even if you don't. I'll go by the library on the way home and see if I can find it."

"That's great, professor," says Joe Zaroom. "I'll sign up. Can I work for pass-fail instead of a grade?"

"Pass-fail?" Roddy laughs, "If you fail, we'll all be your pallbearers."

They each put down some nickels, dimes, and quarters for Violet and move like a flock to Gus at the counter to pay their checks.

"See you next Tuesday."

CHAPTER TWO

STRETCHING LIFE EXPECTANCY TOWARD LIFE SPAN

*V*iolet is there with her order pad. "What will it be today, gentlemen?" She takes their orders and goes to the kitchen. All six cronies had arrived at about the same time, except Lear who had been there long enough to have finished at least one cup of coffee and two cigarettes, the stubs of which had been snuffed out in the little glass ashtray.

"Anything in the paper?" Rodney Thomas asks Lear, who has a newspaper open.

"Naw. Same old stuff, Roddy. Only thing worth reading is the funny paper."

"Well, professor, have you got your lecture prepared?" asks little Joe Zaroom.

"As a matter of fact, I have," Henry says as he draws a small spiral notebook out of his shirt pocket.

"I have learned a lot and there's hope for all of you. The library didn't have a book on the aged Europeans but I found the name of the place they are supposed to live. Abkhazia in the Caucasus Mountains."

"You're a lot of help. What did they do to live so long?"

"Nothing you're going to do. They worked like horses all their lives--climbing up mountains, carrying heavy timbers, farming in primitive ways. One thing I know is there is no way any of you are going to emulate what they did."

"Huh."

"That's the bad news. Now for the good news. They apparently didn't live as long as they said they did. Most researchers who looked at the reports came away with considerable skepticism. Their ages were likely exaggerated."

"That's good news?" Rodney Thomas laughs. "The bad news is we can't do like they do? The good news is they are lying about their ages, anyhow?"

"No, not exactly lying, but inaccurate. But I found this great book while I was looking for the other one. It was written by two Stanford University professors. Let me look at my notes. A good researcher takes careful notes, you know."

Henry still smiles as he licks his thumb and flips a page in his little spiral notebook.

"Age exaggeration seems prevalent, they report, with considerable facts to back them up." Henry then reads: "'It is always possible that the next hidden and exotic society to be investigated will actually have found the secret of long life. But so far, all scientific investigations of claims of great age have failed to confirm the existence of Shangri-La.'"

"Well, Professor, you struck out," says little Joe Zaroom, throwing up his hands. "We're not going to find out how to live forever."

"Not so fast, Zaroom. I'm still up to bat. I found out a lot. At least a lot I didn't know." He thumbs another page in his little notebook. "I found out the difference between 'life span' and 'life expectancy.'"

"Ain't they the same?" Joe asks.

"Life span has been more or less constant for at least a thousand centuries. It is the biological limitation of human life. It is about 100 years, maybe 110. Some say its a little more."

"Sorry, Lear," Roddy says, "that might not be long enough to outlive the Ridenhour brothers."

"I'll take it," says Lear.

"Now life expectancy," Henry continues, "is what, statistically, any one of us here, or all of us as a group, can be expected to live. It is the age when half the people born in a year have died. In ancient Rome it was 22 years, although some of the remaining half might have lived to be a hundred. Life expectancy is the figure insurance companies use when they bet you won't die ahead of your premium schedule."

"So," poses Rodney Thomas, "the life span is the outside limit. Whatever we do, we can't get past that age?"

Will Mack raises his hand, as if in a classroom. "Let me hear you right. Even if medical science finds a cure for all diseases, we can't get past the life span which has been set--or decreed--or whatever? But, . . ."

"That's what I learned from the professors who wrote this book. Life expectancy cannot exceed the life span, but life expectancy for mankind has been expanding constantly."

"Here's what you're saying. We can't get past the life span, but more people are getting a lot closer to it."

"You got it. That is what we want to learn about. We will die within the recognized life span even if all disease is eradicated, even if we do everything to protect our health. This book talks about how to get as close to this outer limit as possible."

"You are saying if we can dodge diseases and jealous husbands, we can make it through to our allotted life span,?" Rodney states. "Why do we die anyhow if there is no accident or disease?"

"As a matter of fact, people do die of something other than disease, or illness, or accident."

"Tell," says Zaroom.

"There's a lot to this book I didn't take notes on," says Henry. "Any of you who want to can go to the library and read the whole thing. Its title is *Vitality and Aging*, by Professors Lawrence Crapo and John Fries. I had the librarian put it on reserve; that means you can read it there but can't check it out. If I were really your professor, I would assign it as homework."

"Thanks for that, professor," says Joe Zaroom. "I'll be satisfied with just what you feed me."

"Tell us how you can die of nothing," asks Will Mack.

"O.K., listen to this from the book: 'What can be the cause of death?' It is the loss of organ reserve. . . ."

"Huh?"

"They explain that scientists are just beginning to understand some additional secrets of human cells, molecules, genes, and how protein is replenished. We know that this complex process keeps the life going in our bodies. We know most of our organs and bodily functions tend to regulate themselves, and to support each other. Jointly they heal injuries and repel invaders, such as unwanted bacteria."

"Go on. What is the nothing that finally kills us?"

"When we are young, our kidneys, the lungs, the heart, along with the other organs, have a considerable reserve. They can do more than they have to do normally to protect us and keep our health in balance. Then they get old and decrepit."

"That's it?" asks Will Mack. "The organs wear out? That is not disease, not illness, and not an accident. You just wear out?"

"That is certainly one theory." Henry looks at his notes. "My authors say, 'The mean level of reserve in many of our organs declines as we grow older.' In time, it follows, the reserve is gone and the capacity is reduced, so we can't fight off the invaders and can't manufacture the replacement substances, and that marks the beginning of the end of the life span."

"You saying it is just going to happen and nothing can be done to increase the life span?" Roddy asks.

"So far that is the way it is and has been. But I suspect a lot more is going to be learned about the aging process itself," Henry answers, "and I am going to look to find out if scientists predict that they can break the life span barrier."

"But not soon enough to help us?"

"Help us? You want to live forever?" asks Roddy.

"What kind of a world would it be if nobody ever died?"

"We would probably kill each other off sooner or later, or we would all starve to death. I don't believe the earth could handle it."

"Maybe we could colonize the planets."

"Well I hope God doesn't have that in mind."

Henry takes charge again. "For all I know, they might find a way to expand the life span. I've gotten into this, and I'll look for that research. Right now our lesson is that cells inevitably wear out, get to the point that they don't regenerate, or do so only slowly. They quit manufacturing proteins, such things as collagen, the stuff that 'holds us together.' Finally, everything wears out, or enough does, so that life cannot be sustained. Either it just ends, or the organ reserve is so diminished that the body cannot resist the environment--a little accident, the heat, the cold, a flu germ."

Lear Jones shifts in his chair and takes a long draw on his cigarette. "That's the final word, Professor? If we are lucky, we just wear out, but there is nothing we can do about it?"

"Oh, no, Henry didn't say there is nothing we can do about it," interrupts Vic Beane. "He says people can live to be a hundred or more, and we need to concentrate now on lasting that long. My lawn mower lasts longer than yours because I keep it in a shed, keep it tuned, and change the oil."

"That's right." Henry wags his finger like a professor. "We can postpone the time when we wear out. We have to accept, with the knowledge scientists now have, that there is a finite life span for human beings, and we do not fully understand why this is so, nor why it has been about the same for 100,000 years, nor whether it can be lengthened. You got that right. Even if we get past accidents and disease and illness, we wear out, and we can't help wearing out. Beanie is also right. With a little luck, and a little trying, we can avoid wearing out before our time. That's what we need to talk about."

Beane interrupts, visibly excited. "I know there are some things we can do to keep our blood vessels from wearing out so soon. What are they? I drain out my garden hose, and hang it in the shed in the winter, and I've been using it since Eisenhower was President. I do more for my garden equipment than I do for myself. If we are going to wear out, regardless, surely we can learn ways to keep organs stronger, longer"

"Stronger, longer. That's what they say."

"I paint my house every ten years or so," Vic continues. "I bought my house right after World War II. It was built in the thirties. Henry's company is getting ready to replace all the electrical wiring. I've already repaired and replaced the plumbing. It's better than new. Theoretically, it will never wear out. Can't we do things to keep our lungs, liver, other organs in top condition?"

"Sounds easy," Rodney cuts in, "but Henry's company can't re-wire your body, and transplanting a new plumbing system sounds unreal. If you had to stick with your old wires and pipes and paint, your house would already be gone."

"Transplants?"

"Who knows?"

"Where would you get them--if everybody is going to stop dy-ing. . . ?"

"All right, students, let's have a little order." Henry raises his finger and his voice. He is obviously enjoying his classroom.

"I am not halfway through my notes. Let's work our way up to what we can do, Victor. Let's get back to the book. One step at a time. They tell us that infectious diseases--smallpox, tuberculosis, typhus, and measles, and so on--have all but been eliminated. Flu and pneumonia deaths have been reduced to about 15 percent of what they were in 1900."

"So people have to find something else to die from," laughs Roddy.

"Yes, you might say that, but first," Henry says in his true pro-fessorial tone, "let's consider what are the ways people die before they approach the end of the life span? The charts show automo-biles kill far too many people.

"Many more than in 1900," grins Roddy.

"For sure, and we don't have figures on 1900 deaths from run-away horses. But most older people die from chronic diseases--cardiovascular disorders, cancer, and strokes, and several others, all of which have greatly increased in this century. This increase, the book's authors say, is because we have virtually eliminated infec-tious diseases."

"Yes, modern science has caught the infectious diseases, but" asks Beane, "haven't the demands of modern life unduly stressed the heart and the nervous system?"

"Stress!" Old Lear perks up." "Modern Life! We don't have any stress like they had when I was born. Seventy, eighty years ago you had to chop your firewood for your cookstove. Had to worry about old age and no money. Wasn't no Social Security. Had to walk to find a phone to get a doctor when your baby was burning up with diphtheria fever, and he came by buggy or Model-T Ford. Everything is easier now. I remember my childhood--the stress and strain of daily life my parents went through. Modern life, modern kids! Let them quit bitching."

Vic Beane, the grandson of a slave, reminded, nods in agreement. "Excuse my foolishness, Lear."

"What Henry is telling us, Vic," says Rodney. "You don't die earlier from something else, infectious diseases, so more people live on to face the ultimate killers that were out there lying in wait all the time?"

"Not a bad tradeoff," says Joe Zaroom.

"And if you can miss the killers," asks Will Mack, "then the question is, how to wear out as slowly as possible."

"Right, and that means we need to know about preserving organ reserve.

"You're on target, and while I think of it," says Henry, "let me interject a new thought. I was reading about the mortality of regular cells and I came across a fascinating fact. Cancer cells, most types, are apparently immortal. That means they will live and reproduce forever in a test tube. Normal human cells will reproduce only about fifty times. I am going to follow up on that and see what I can find. I don't know the lesson in that for us but one of these days scientists are going to solve the riddle of life. I think, not too many years from now, medical science will be able to stop cancer in its tracks and as a by-product we will learn from that how to slow down the aging process, maybe how to increase the reproduction of healthy cells. Fascinating." Henry looks stern and serious.

Will Mack interrupts. "Great! But I don't want to lose our focus. Go back with me a minute. You are saying that there is presently no known way to expand the life span of humans, but that we do know how to get further along that life span than most have been getting? So, how do we stretch out our lives toward the end of the life span?"

Henry smiles. "Back to page 67. We can indeed stretch toward the life span. Let's look at the villains. Let me quote: 'Acute infectious illnesses and their huge contribution to the mortality and morbidity rates are nearly gone. . . . Now our society must find ways to meet the challenges of chronic illness.'"

"Chronic illness? How can we sidestep them? You mentioned that in passing," says Will Mack.

"Not in passing. That is our question for discussion, gentlemen. How do we reach old age? How? First, by avoiding the chronic illnesses. The authors refer to them as 'universal diseases.' Cardiovascular, cancer, strokes, are the prevalent ones, but we will consider other chronic illnesses? How do we hold them off? Can we? That is our question. I'll get to that at the next class--the next breakfast, that is."

"Avoid disease? That's all?"

"No, not all. Along with that, how do we keep our vital organs as vital as possible? Those are the two fundamental questions--the hopes of longer life."

"Okay," says Victor. "The two goals: Avoid chronic diseases. Protect, keep healthy, the vital organs."

"You got it. How to avoid chronic disease? How to keep vital organs strong? That is what we need to know."

Henry closes his little spiral notebook, and puts it back in his shirt pocket.

"That's it. It is time to go. Roddy has got to pretend he is working. I've got to go to the grocery store to get some eggs and coffee.

"Now next Friday I will have some more for you, and I am going to have to look at some other books to find out how to live longer in good health -- if any of you want to come back. And Gus will be serving breakfast as usual."

"Great, Henry, see you Friday."

"Home run!" says Joe Zaroom.

They put change on the table for Violet. Two or three take quick sips of water. All crowd up the aisle by the counter seats to Gus Tukuras at the cash register.

Chapter Three

SLOW DOWN THE KILLERS. GO OUT SWINGING!

*T*he morning comes dimly through a slight rainfall. Henry looks at his inside-outside thermometer. He has on his wrinkled pajama bottoms.

Hum, not springtime after all. Down at least ten degrees.

Henry never could wait for Gus's coffee. He puts two measuring spoons of coffee into the percolator, and fills it with water to the proper line. He plugs in the cord to the pot, and then plugs it into the outlet.

Funny how many little safety precautions you learn in a lifetime, he muses to himself. *I know how to plug in a coffee pot. Can't say I haven't learned anything in seventy-two years.*

Little precautions, thousands of them, make older people less accident prone. That's what the statistics say. It's the young who get killed in accidents. I drive more carefully. I fasten my seatbelt--most of the time. I'm just more careful.

Let me count the other things. We don't leave an obstacle course of shoes and clutter between our bed and the bathroom. I keep a free hand on the rail side when using stairs. I don't start across the street if it appears I'll have to run to beat a car. I use a slip-proof mat in the shower. We've done away with throw rugs that slip.

Henry puts the coffee can back on the shelf.

Yet old people still have a hazard because they get forgetful. Already I am. How many times has Lottie reminded me--nagged me--about forgetting to cut off the oven? Think! I let my mind wander too much. I'm thinking of what I want to do about so many things. Pay attention! No wonder old people are forgetful; there is so much yet to be done; there is so much to clutter one's mind.

"But, hell, I'm not old." He slaps his hand on the counter, rattles the percolator.

Henry hurriedly dashes barefooted for his newspaper, but does not go look at his plants. He gets an old tan raincoat out of the closet by the front door, and lays it on a chair. Then he walks back to the bathroom and plugs in his electric razor.

Shortly he is back in the kitchen, fully dressed. He has on a gray, smartly-pressed suit, and a dark red tie.

He looks out the kitchen window. *Gosh, I shouldn't wear a suit just back from the cleaners on a day like this. Oh, well.*

He pours his second mug of coffee, walks back to the front door, sipping as he goes, pulls on his raincoat, steps out the front door and shuts it quietly and firmly. He dashes to his car, some dozen feet from the stoop, jumps in and slides his hand across his forehead to dissipate the raindrops. He wears no hat. He places the coffee mug on the dashboard, creating a patch of fog on the windshield, and searches in his coat pocket for the keys. He sticks the key in the switch, takes a sip of coffee, then turns the key and cranks the four-year old Chevrolet. It whirs and then chokes. He takes another sip of coffee. He turns the switch again and the motor races and then calms to a regular beat.

Henry shifts into gear, takes the wheel in his left hand, the coffee in his right, and sips as the seat belt buzzer sounds its allotted time and then gives up and quits.

Downtown Henry notes three cars parked in front of the U.S. Grill with plenty of spaces on each side. Parking, he slams the door and trots to the cafe door, rushing in.

"Why did you let it rain, Gus?" he calls as he pulls off his coat and brushes his hand across his hair.

"Can't help it on Fridays, Mr. Henry. Besides, it's good for the crops."

"That it is." Henry makes his way to the rear table. Lear Jones, Victor Beane, and Rodney Thomas are there sipping coffee. From ashtray evidence, Lear has finished two cigarettes.

"Morning, boys!"

Gus's kitchen always has good smells, especially so on a rainy morning, and odors of frying bacon and potatoes and well-toasted bread warm the restaurant. Henry sits down as Violet brings him a cup of coffee.

"Great day, Violet," Henry greets her.

"Sure is. Glad I'm not a traffic cop or a garbage collector."

Victor Beane takes a sip of coffee, and with fingers extended wags his hand rhythmically as if he were counting boxcars. "Henry," he says to the beat of his hand, "I've been thinking about something you said yesterday."

He puts his hands, palms down by his coffee cup. "This business of organ reserve getting so slight that you just pass on, die, without any illness, doesn't add up. Your defenses are just so weak that any old germ can get through and finish you off. You can't just die. You die from something. The germ kills you."

"That makes some sense. But Doctors Crapo and Fries report that some people just lie down and die."

Victor shakes his head. "So nobody cares much about the cause when that happens. They don't perform an autopsy. They don't look for the villain. But something caused the system to stop. Do doctors put 'old age' as the cause of death on the death certificate? Is that a legal cause?"

"I don't know, Beanie. It seems possible that the old machinery just quits. I suppose we don't need to know what the doctors wrote to agree that the aging process cannot be stopped, that aging is inexorable, that we cannot, whatever steps we take, live beyond a certain age."

"Maybe I don't want to admit that, intellectually," Beane mumbles.

Henry continues. "Intellectually? Now what is the point of knowing that? Acceptance of aging is the beginning of wisdom about aging. We can't avoid getting old, aging, but we can do two things, and neither is more important than the other.

As Victor and Henry are so intently talking, Joe Zaroom and Will Mack come in, shuffle into their chairs, and receive their coffee from Violet. And there stands Violet with her order pad folded back, pencil poised for action. Henry ignores the interruption and Violet.

"First there are numerous ways to minimize the chances of contracting one of the chronic diseases that plague older people," Henry continues. "Luck is involved, to be sure, but we can add to our luckiness.

"Second, we can slow down our own rate of aging, and come a little closer, close as possible, to the maximum human life span, and more important as far as I am concerned, we can hope that when we finally run out of organ reserve we will be in good health--not crippled with disease, that is--and happy, and self-dependent. Then when it is time to die we can get on with it without hanging around as an invalid. We die a natural death, as the book calls it."

"Yea," Joe chimes in. "We are not taking age as a teammate. We are breaking a tackle, continuing to run."

"Fair enough" nods Henry.

Rodney sits back in his chair. "The ideal, you are saying, is that if we do certain positive things, we might very well go the last few miles on our own feet instead of in a wheel chair or an invalid's bed."

"If we are lucky," says Joe Zaroom.

"Sure," says Henry, "but it's not all luck. We can do something about it! That is the point--or an important one--of studying the aging process."

"I accept that. How do we go out swinging?" Victor takes his hands off the table and leans back.

"Right! Okay, Violet,!" commands Henry, snapping his fingers.

"Yes sir, capitaine!" Violet strikes a pose of military attention.

As Violet is writing down the orders, a man approaches the table, wearing a tailored dark pinstripe suit with a vest. He has thick dark brown hair firmly slicked back, black horn-rimmed glasses, trim figure, shirt collar held by a silver pin, sliding gracefully as if he were moving without lifting his feet.

"John McCorn!" exclaims Henry. "Where have you been so long?"

"Johnny!"

Lear raises his hand in a peace-be-with-you salute as the others greet the visitor. "John Boy!"

As John passes Violet, he imperceptibly rubs her chubby buttocks. She cuts her eyes toward him but keeps on writing.

"I am truly sorry I have not been here, friends." McCorn speaks rapidly, words rushing like water from a hose. "I have to make a living, you know. Unlike you rich and retired people. But you know I never...."

"Say rich *or* retired," drawls Lear.

"Henry, I am so delighted you are talking about aging. A fascinating subject. I was so excited when Roddy told me. I am so sorry I have missed it. It is a privilege to be sitting at your feet and learning, as I have been doing ever since I was a boy. I can't...."

Lear cuts him off. "How's your business?" .

"Famous. Just famous. Violet, may I have a cup of tea, please?" John winks at her. His voice is pleasant, but high-powered.

"Why not? Everybody else drinks coffee."

John smiles at her and turns to Henry. "Now, Henry, I am dieting, taking vitamins, jogging three times a week when I can, quit smoking and strong drink--or some of it, and am dyeing my hair. What else do I do to live forever?"

"You missed the first lesson," says Will Mack. "You can't live forever no matter what you do."

"That is a good place for me to take out my notebook," says Henry.

Henry, still sipping coffee, opens his little notebook. "I'm hooked. I've started looking for other books in the library. Research in aging is not an old science, so it is good enough for me to start our review about 1960. Two books I've found as a good starting point are the *Handbook of Aging and the Individual* (1959), edited by James E. Birren, with lots of articles, and Alex Comfort's *Ageing: The Biology of Senescence*, which was revised and republished in 1964."

Zaroom interrupts. "What's a 'Senescence'?"

"That's a fancy word for aging, British influence, just like they spell aging with an 'e.' That book is by Alex Comfort, an early leader in geriatric research, who is British."

"I want 'senescence' on my death certificate," says Joe. "But not too soon."

"I'll speak to the coroner for you, Joe, but let me sum up for John. This is not a graduate course. I cite these two textbooks for those who want to find out more about such subjects as aging of birds and fish, and other research subjects. I read them, or most of them, to get myself a foundation for the whole problem.

"Comfort put it right when he wrote that the 'assignment' of biology in the study of old age is to devise if possible a means of keeping human beings alive in active health for a longer time than would normally be the case--in other words, 'to prolong individual life.'

"I am looking for reports of scientific studies and experiments in order to know what I am talking about. We can't start studying if we don't understand what the aging process is. Then we need to know what we can do about it."

Roddy adds, "What is happening to make us grow old? And how do we handle it?"

"Right, and then we get down to specifics. First, what are the chronic diseases and ailments that especially attack older people?"

"And what we can do to avoid them."

"You've got it. Actually, John, I was reviewing a book written by two Stanford University doctors. I was just hitting the highlights.

"Let's see, we were told that the medical profession has all but eliminated the infectious diseases--from measles and mumps to dyptheria and scarlet fever,--so not many of us are going to die from them.

"Now, next, there are a lot of other things that can kill us or cripple us or make us wish we were dead.

"We do not know fully how to avoid all those dangers. For example, we can't avoid getting cancer in the same way we can avoid breaking a leg on a ski slope. We can stay away from the skis, but we don't know what all to stay away from to keep from getting cancer."

"So, John," says Rodney, "we first want to know enough to dodge a lot of the diseases of old age."

"Tell you what, John, why don't you just buy the book? It is worth keeping. You can read it in those motel rooms if you ever find time from your price charts. It is called *Vitality and Aging.*

"You will get a kick out of their one-hoss shay metaphor carried throughout the book. Like the one-hoss shay--if we live right, and are lucky, we just one day wear out all over and are gone.

"Sounds interesting. Reckon Intimate Book Store has it?"

"Probably. I haven't begun to tell all that is in the book, John. I haven't begun to cite all the proof and advice the scholars have arrayed. I have just given us a quick review, with one main conclusion I have drawn."

"Roll on, Henry. I never thought we could live forever. We're talking about living longer. Right, Will Mack?"

"That's right, John," Victor Beane says. "And healthier, which I think is more important than longer. We want to dodge the many chronic diseases that cripple a lot of senior citizens."

"And the good news," says Henry, "is that, knowing all this, there are many things we can do to arrest, delay, or avoid these chronic, or universal, diseases."

"Now there's the nut in the peanut," says Zaroom.

Henry flips to the back of his little notebook. "So you will know, after we finish chronic diseases, I am going to try to find some facts about non-fatal illnesses that slow down older people, and various disabilities that strike older people."

"See John," says Zaroom. "We've got a whole semester ahead of us."

"All right, Professor. Tell how to avoid the veritable chronic log trucks," says Roddy.

"First, I have written down part of one paragraph I think we need to understand. I told you the authors suggested *universal* disease is a more apt term than *chronic* disease--meaning everybody is subject to have them. Now listen to this," says Henry, reading very deliberately, spacing out each word, "' . . . we suggest that more important insights come from the fact that these diseases tend to, one, be incremental, two, be universal, three, have a clinical threshold, and four, be characterized by a progressive loss of organ reserve.'"

"You'll have to read it three or four more times for it to sink in through my thick skull. What does it mean?" asks Roddy.

"Well, you know what they mean by *universal*. Everybody is vulnerable. I suppose you could say everybody has at least a trace of these diseases."

"Understood," nods Will Mack. "Proceed."

"Now consider their word incremental." Henry unconsciously reverts to his professorial tone. "*Incremental*. These universal diseases begin early in adulthood, gradually doing a little damage and then a little more, cutting at you relentlessly, if slowly, so you are getting worse or more susceptible by increments every day. You can imagine the vessels getting a little more brittle, a little more clogged. These chronic or universal diseases tend to be incremental."

"Damn," says Lear, "they've been eating on me all my life and I didn't ever know it."

"That's right," adds Rodney. "The goo starts clinging to your arteries, according to my doctor, when you eat your first egg and sausage and keeps on until there is no place for the blood to flow."

"Ugh--not so graphic."

"Well, now," Henry says, as if calling a class back to order, "that is the important point. If you know these diseases are gaining on you every day, then you can understand that you might be able to do something every day to slow them down."

"Well, what can weak, lazy, procrastinating human beings do?" Victor asks.

"Much, and we'll get to that."

First, think about the two other things I read to you. These diseases have a *clinical threshold*. That means, while proceeding incrementally, one day you will wake up with the disease at the clinical, identifiable, diagnosable level."

"'Boom, says the doctor, you have a heart attack," Will Mack strikes his fist into the air. "Or emphysema--or lung cancer--or a stroke--which has been creeping up on you all these years."

"Right. The point is that you don't get a stroke all at once. The clinical threshold is when you know it."

"Well, I follow that, I do believe," said Will Mack. "And what we want to do is to hold back the threshold as long as possible? Or never reach it at all? Right?"

"Certainly that's the reason for knowing these conditions are incremental."

"Yeh," says Rodney, "It's a cinch--get rid of a lifetime of bad habits. I am reminded of the story of the frontier man who, limping in with heart problems, was told by his doctor to give up whiskey and red meat, or he would die. He couldn't handle the thought. He immediately got a jug of likker and a two-pound T-bone steak, ate, drank--and, before morning, died."

Henry frowns, but the other four laugh. "You will remember that I read that this universal, incremental path toward the clinical threshold of chronic diseases is marked by a progressive *loss of organ reserve*. The capacity of all of your organs, immune systems, and nervous systems are getting a little more worn every year, every day, less able to protect you from the chronic, universal diseases creeping closer every day toward the clinical threshold."

"So," interjects Will Mack, "we want to slow the incremental advance of the universal diseases to avoid reaching the threshold, and slow down the wearing out or loss of reserve of the body's organs?"

"Simply and clearly put," answers Henry.

"The question is how."

"Exactly, that's the name of this course."

Rodney Thomas stands up. "My rear end reserve is exhausted. Time to go!"

"You've got a point, Roddy. But hold a minute! Let me sum up by mentioning my fourth point-- loss of organ reserve. This is something we need to know: What can we do to protect as long as possible our organ reserve? That may be our biggest challenge."

"Well start with what causes our organs to age? Does it have to happen?" asks Victor.

"It seems the scientists are a long way from understanding the life cycle of vital organs. I'm looking for some answers, Beanie. In the meantime, gentlemen, what is your pleasure?"

"Give us some more, Henry," says Will Mack.

"Right on," adds Joe Zaroom. "Find out about exercise. How can we keep running the bases?"

"I know I ought to quit something," Lear says. "Whiskey?"

Roddy is standing. "Henry, I worry that I am going to lose my wits, get senile. How do you dodge that bullet?"

"I'll look into that," says Henry.

"Henry," John McCorn puts his hand on Henry's shoulder. "Before you go. You said you had one main conclusion. What is it?"

"Simple. All of us can live a whole lot longer than we think we can." Roddy turns to go. The others start to get up.

"Wait," says Victor. "I want to tell you something. I've been thinking all morning how to get this into the conversation. Give me just a minute."

"Sure," says Henry.

"I went out to the Lullaby Rest Home yesterday. Wimpy and old Fireball Jackson and Billy Diason are there. I've been meaning to go. Put it off. Conscience bothered me. I went. Wish I hadn't. Glad I did.

"Wimpy was in a wheel chair. Wouldn't let go when we shook hands. Just stared at me. Such sad eyes.

"I talked to him about the times we used to go hunting. He never said a word. Vegetable soup was dried and clotted all over his pajama lap. Little pieces of carrots and butter beans. I talked to him a while, then patted him on the shoulder and left. He recognized me, I know. He was so sad.

"They told me I couldn't see Fireball, that he was confined to his bed, but I found him anyhow. He was confined, all right, in spades. He was naked and two big belts like a mule's bellyband had him tied down, couldn't move his arms. There was an un-made bed in the other corner of the room, terrible stench. As soon as he saw me, he yelled, 'Victor, get me out of this hell hole.' I tried to calm him down and he told me he had called the head lady a thieving son-of-a-bitch.

"I laughed and told him that was one thing he shouldn't have called a lady, but he didn't think it was funny. He said she blew a whistle and three big men, one the janitor, came running in and threw him to the floor, and he wrestled and fought and they dragged him to his room tearing off his pajamas. They got him in bed, him fighting all the time, and buckled him in. I asked him when it happened and he said early that morning. He was steaming mad.

"I got down under the bed and unbuckled him. He got up and went to the bathroom. He came back with a towel around him and sat in the chair and I sat on the side of the bed. He said he got mad when he found out what they charged him for medicine when he wasn't getting anything but aspirin and sleeping tablets. He said he shouldn't have lost his temper, but he did, and she didn't give him a chance to talk about it.

"We talked for an hour. He wants out. I told him I would talk to his daughter, and I took the two belts and threw them out of the hall window.

"I wandered around and found Billy by himself in a little room with eight or ten chairs, watching television, a children's cartoon show, just sitting there. He was really glad to see me. He was alert and bright and the first thing I did was to laugh and ask him why he was watching that stuff. He said they weren't allowed to change channels, only the attendants could do that, and he had been hoping one would come by. I switched it to an old movie.

"I cut it off.

"We talked a long time about old times, and I asked him how he was doing, how things were at home. It tore me up. He said, 'I don't know what I have done to deserve to end up my life in prison. We are not human beings here, but that's the way it is. I can't do anything about it. I've got cancer of the prostate, spread considerable, and I'm not going to live much longer, and I don't have any money left, just Medicaid, and I don't have any family left. I just put up with all this but it hurts me so to see the way they treat people, like they are nothing.

"I couldn't stand it any longer. I told Billy I'd be back to see him next week, and left.

"I don't do much crying. I remember my grandpa saying to me before I ever started school, 'Boys don't cry.' I don't know why that is, but he said it and I believed it. He musta had plenty of chances to cry in his hard boyhood.

"I came out of that nursing home with lumps swelling up in my stomach and chest and got in my car and started up and found myself bawling. I was crying, crying so loud I could hear it, not just whimpering or shedding a little tear.

"I was crying, and it was a shock to me. What's happening, I asked myself. I've never done this in my life. Those poor people, imprisoned by sickness and poverty, ignored and neglected, forgotten, at the end that will not end.

"I was depressed, really depressed, I realized. I was mad. I was distressed. But why was I crying? Boys don't cry. I was crying for those pitiful friends, but I knew also I was crying for my own fears as much as for their sadness. That scared me.

"Well, that won't do, I said to myself. We've got to change things, we've got to get them out, all of them, not just our friends. I'm not going to end up in that condition. I'll rise above it. I'll keep my independence. Maybe--and maybe I can't control fate.

"Then I pulled my car to the shoulder and stopped, and slapped the steering wheel. Right now I'll go more often to help them through their last lonely sadness, I told myself. I'll raise hell about their treatment. I'll take the mayor out there. I'll take Alton from the newspaper. I'll get on Charlie to do something in Washington about Medicaid.

"Then I slapped the wheel again, and drove off and said, 'Snap out of it, Victor. Boys don't cry.'

Victor leans back in his chair.

"Thank you, Victor," says Will Mack, "you've got a volunteer. We have all been blind to the way old people are treated."

"Let's get organized," says Joe.

Chapter Four

JUST FOUR THINGS TO REMEMBER

*V*iolet is taking away the dirty dishes. Henry backs up his chair and says, "Let's take up where we left off. I have now looked at a dozen other books, and I'll refer to them as we go along. We were beginning to talk about the chronic diseases."

"Henry," says Roddy, "I asked about losing my wits, when it would happen, how would I know? This morning I was out of the house and into my car before I realized I had forgot to put on my belt. I'm losin' it, Henry. Are you going to talk about senility?"

"That's not old age," says Will Mack. "When I was in high school I went to a dance and realized in the middle of the first dance that my britches were falling off. I had forgotten my belt and was frantically trying to hitch them up while dancing with one hand on my date when she asked what was happening and took charge. She had three little ribbons in her hair and took one of them and drew my two back belt loops together with a bow knot. I was holding up my coat and she was kneeling down behind me when Hambone Lewis saw this little scene and yelled, 'Stop the music!' Then they all gathered 'round and watched her finish the job. They kidded me for years. If I were to run into Hambone today, he'd mention it first thing. She was one sweet thing and I thought she would make a wonderful bride. But she moved off to Milwaukee. You'll be all right, Roddy."

Whoa," says Henry, "We were going to talk about chronic dis-eases. We'll talk about belts when I can find the right book."

"Where is Hambone, now?" asks Rodney.

"I've lost track of him. He ought to be in the penitentiary."

Henry says, "I don't think you've lost it yet, Roddy. Now, let's start with cancer. This is our most frightening foe. There are so many kinds. The causes are known, suspected, and unknown.

"These are your chronic or universal diseases?" asks Will Mack.

"Yes, and for cancer, our best hope is the continuing research that is being done. We may learn what triggers cancer.

"In the meantime, what can older people do?"

Rodney raised his hand. "I don't mean to be frivolous in the face of such a serious matter, but I cut out this article, waiting for just this chance. What can older people do? Let me read it to you.

"It is from the April 10, 1989 issue of *Insight*.

"Dr. Joe D. Wassersug was listening to the conversation be-tween two octogenarian doctors who conclude that the preferred way to die is by massive heart attacks and strokes. He was startled. He thought, I've been living wrong! My problem is that I am too healthy. My blood pressure and cholesterol levels are normal, and I don't smoke. I am unlikely to die that way. 'What else is left to terminate my existence? *Cancer*? Horrible! Perish the thought.' He writes. 'I resolved to take a more active intervention in my destiny. I scanned the menu and ordered the thickest slab of rare beef. . . . If a fat enriched, high cholesterol gourmet diet can prevent death from cancer, I say it's worth it. Pass the butter, please.'"

Henry laughs. "That is probably as good a strategy as the next. But I don't believe I'll try it. It would be my luck to be laid up with a stroke for ten years. So let me talk about cancer.

"We have two shots at cancer--until the researchers find out more of the secrets--defensive action, and early discovery with prompt treatment.

"Cancer is when cells are in revolt--unrestrained in multiplica-tion, attacking, and invading neutral territories. I have great faith that science will discover the flaw that causes such behavior. They are delving into the secrets of DNA, genetic engineering, and life itself. But whatever causes cancer, we do not want to trigger the villain. We don't want to prompt the revolt of the cells.

"Now," asks Rodney, "how do we hunker down, dig the fox holes, fortify the high ground to repel the attack?"

"A number of things, the experts say. A few general rules. Don't try to win any suntanning contests. Skin cancer.

"Cut down on fatty foods and eat more roughage. Colon cancer. Nutrition makes a difference, and I'll find out a little more about that.

"Limit alcohol. You asked about that Lear. Bad on your liver, for one thing. Don't smoke. You didn't ask about that Lear. But quit!

"Now there is something about damage from metabolism--the use of foods--free radicals--but I will have to search for more about that.

"The next, very important thing you can do, is to keep a close eye on yourself. Self-examination for early symptoms, changing moles or birthmarks or growths. Bumps. Nodules. Blood in stools. If you are suspicious, see your doctor. Don't put it off.

"Next, a cancer propensity may be in your genes. In your family history. Have a routine medical exam every year--especially for colon cancer and for prostate cancer.

"Women should pay careful attention for signs of breast cancer, cancer of the cervix, and should, every several years, have a mammogram and other appropriate tests."

"But," says Rodney, "they are saying that the mammogram triggers cancer in some women, because of a peculiar gene."

"I saw that account, but so far it has not been pinned down. I'd say a woman should ask her doctor. This is a cutting-edge discovery, identifying particular genes."

"Yes, but it says radiation treatment might prompt more cancer."

"Yes, well it is a worry, but it also shows they are getting to the secrets of the genes. She should consult with her doctor."

"Henry, have we left out something?" asks Will Mack. "Doesn't keeping the organ reserve up have something to do with warding off all diseases?"

"No doubt about it. Last point, stay trim. Good for all ailments."

"And luck," adds Joe Zaroom.

Victor Beane claps his hands. "Now that ought not to be too hard!"

Roddy says, "No, not hard at all. Impossible! I can handle the self-examination and maybe go to the doctor. But staying trim! I'm already losing that battle."

"Murphy, I see a damnable pattern coming out of all this," says Lear. "Clean living! Maybe we ought to chuck all this study right now."

Henry smiles and sips his coffee, "I've just begun, just touched on only one of the chronic, universal diseases. I've next got the heart and the brain to go."

"Henry," says Victor, "Do any of those things really ward off cancer? If so, why? Why should exercise, staying trim, have anything to do with cancer? It's in your genes. You can't catch it, but you can't head it off, I'd think."

"I hope to find something about your body's immune system and we will see what we can learn. I can tell you what I think. It is a matter of keeping fit. Your body has a lot to do with keeping you well. Your body can maybe nip a wild cancer cell in the bud. Your body repairs cells that might otherwise turn into cancer. Not always, of course. It stands to reason that your body reserves generally are kept healthier if you are healthy."

"What about free radicals," asks Victor. "How does that cause cancer?" What is it?"

"I've just found a book and I will find out more about free radicals. Free radicals apparently do a lot of damage. Cancer. Organ reserve. Cell distortion."

"But luck plays a big part, I'd say. Cancer just happens. You can't get vaccinated," says Joe.

"It's luck, Joe, but you can load the dice. For one thing, smoking, they have proved can cause cancer."

"Hasn't caught Lear yet."

"Tough genes," says Lear.

"And the caution about fats and roughage has to do with colon cancer, among other things," says Victor Beane. "I reckon all that makes sense."

"Cancer's scary," says Joe. "Like walking home at night. Some punk might just up and shoot you."

"But you don't have to walk at night, Joe," says Rodney. "Certainly not alone."

"Right. You can't avoid cancer for sure," Henry continues. "We don't yet know enough about it. So examine yourself and get examined--at first suspicion. A great many kinds of cancer can be treated and cured."

"You said you are coming back to nutrition. Surely getting the right nutrients has something to do with punching all the little buttons and pulling all the little levers in the body's immune mechanisms, which keep the vital organs, the cells, and everything else running right. We've heard about antioxidants, vitamins, trace elements. . . ."

"No doubt about it, Will. I'll keep at this, and find more about nutrients, antioxidants and free radicals, and vitamins. Let me get back right now to the next chronic disease."

Rodney raises his hand, "Henry, staying in shape may apply to all illnesses. All these precautions may not be as numerous as they sound. There's a lot of overlap. When you get through scaring us with all the illnesses, and killing all our pleasures, let's collate the precautions. We might be able to handle it."

"Good idea. Now, let me go to the other big killer. Cardiovascular illnesses. The cardiovascular diseases--the heart and the blood vessels--strokes and heart disease. This includes a lot of subheads. Heart disease, first. More people have arthritis than any other ailment of the old, but more people go to the hospital, and to the grave, because of heart diseases.

"The major cause of heart disease is arteriosclerosis, the hardening of the arteries and blockage of the blood flow, and its most frequent form is atherosclerosis, which is plaque accumulated on the inner walls of the blood vessels, mostly at or near the heart."

"Take us slowly. What is 'plaque?'"

"A combination of stuff, but mostly cholesterol, which builds up inside blood vessels, and in time can block them. That's atherosclerosis--cuts off blood, that is oxygen and nutrients, to the heart muscle."

"Slows down the blood the heart is pumping?"

"No, this blood is not going directly into the heart chamber, where blood is pumped to the lungs for oxygen and then back again. You should know that the heart muscle doesn't get its oxygen and nutrients from blood going through the chambers of the heart, but by three main coronary blood vessels on the outside of the heart, which in turn have further branches. It is in these where the mischief is done when they are hardened or blocked. We are talking about the blood in the vessels that nourish the cells of the heart muscle, like it nourishes the muscles such as your biceps."

"So the blood that is blocked is the blood nourishing the pump?"

"You've got it. This shortage of nutrients and oxygen damages the heart muscle, actually can kill some of the cells. 'Infarct' means dead tissue. You have heard that someone suffered myocardial infarction. Myocardial refers to the heart muscle. Death of some heart muscle."

"I see," says Vic. "The blood is on the outside of the heart, keeping the heart muscle nourished, so the blockage starves and damages the heart muscle?"

"You got it. Now, another word to remember is thrombus, which is a clot of blood, and thrombosis is the forming of a clot. It is a heart attack when the clot gets jammed in a vessel close to the heart which has been narrowed by atherosclerosis. If oxygen and nutrients are cut off or cut down, the heart can't handle it, and that is a heart attack."

"How do you know you have an attack?" asks Victor.

"I once asked my doctor how I could tell the difference between pain from indigestion and pain from heart trouble. He said, 'You'll know!'

"But Senator David Pryor of Arkansas, who happens to be the chairman of the U.S. Senate Committee on Aging, has a better answer for your question, Beanie. He had a heart attack. He recovered and wrote about it in a magazine, *Arkansas Times* (August 1991). I clipped it. Let me read. 'I had bolted upward in bed and looked at the clock--1:45 a.m. I was lying in a pool of perspiration, soaked from head to toe. My upper chest did not feel sharp pain, but some-

thing better described as massive discomfort. Could it be indigestion? Did I really eat a live porcupine? Within minutes . . . the in-
tensity of the pain increased. . . . I'm getting light headed I
knew I was having a heart attack. . . . I reached for the phone and
punched 9-1-1. . . . My chest tightened. My rib cage became a vice. I
was losing consciousness. . . . I do remember being helped onto a
stretcher. Inside the ambulance . . . the woman attendant asked me,
"From one to ten, how much pain are you having?" I held up ten
fingers.'

"Like the doctor said, you'll know, and I have a publication of
the National Institutes of Health. Says the pain may spread to
shoulders, arms, and neck, maybe the back, and you may suffer
nausea, sweating, and shortage of breath, and feel weak.

"The pain will be 'vise-like, or constricting, as if a rope were
being pulled tightly around the chest.' "

"Right," says Joe. "That's 'The Big One,' as Fred Sanford of Sanford and Son called it."

"I reckon. But don't stand around clowning. A heart attack calls
for you to go--to be taken that is--immediately to the hospital in a
prone position--immediately. The first thing David Pryor did was
dial 9-1-1, and was rushed to the hospital. You can't wait around
for it to go away."

"You said Senator Pryor recovered, Henry. What are the odds?"
asks Victor.

"I'd say good if prompt treatment is obtained. The means of
treatment are getting better all the time, but I'll not go into all of
that, because I didn't bargain to give you a medical education. We
want to know what we can do to keep from having a heart attack in
the first place.

"The grim fact is that over a third of the people who have a
heart attack don't get a chance at rehabilitation. So don't delay."

"We don't even want to be in the two-thirds," says Rodney.
"What all causes heart attacks? How do we ward them off?"

"Okay. Remember that a crucial blood vessel gets clogged. One
advance red flag is the amount of cholesterol in your blood. There
are other warnings--chest pains and shortage of breath when exercising, or when just walking, or frequent fatigue. Your physician

can, where indicated, get a pretty accurate view of the clogging with catheterization--running a tube through a blood vessel from your leg or arm to your heart--and taking an angiogram, an x-ray picture. Dye in the blood reveals the blockages--maybe while you are undergoing a stress test."

Rodney interrupts Henry: "I asked my doctor to give me this catheter test, after my cousin had a triple bypass, and he refused. Said it was risky. Said he already knew enough about my heart."

"Of course. It is fairly risky and not for casual use. You have a long record of medical exams. Your doctor listens to your heart with a stethoscope, takes your blood pressure, takes your electro-cardiogram--an EKG--counts your pulse, may x-ray your heart, or take an echogram, and a number of other procedures. You already have a medical record, and a regular physical exam, as your doctor suggests, is the way to get advance notice about a possible heart attack."

"It's good to know about the advance notice," says Rodney. "But how do we keep a clean bill of health?"

"Yeah, I want to know about that," says Will Mack, "but before we leave the doctor's office, what about bypass surgery? Is it safe now? When is it necessary? Is it used too often, perhaps when not needed?"

"I am reading here," Henry answers, "that coronary bypass is a fairly recent development, but the operation is now almost routine. So it is safe--although there is risk to any operation.

"The bypass procedure is to remove a large vein from the leg and use it to replace the blocked or damaged blood vessels that nourish the heart.

"These operations are not for everyone, although in this NIH booklet Dr. Levy tells us that those 'who were once incapacitated and limited to low-level activity can generally be relieved of pain with this procedure. There is also evidence that coronary bypass surgery in properly selected patients improved the function of the left ventricle or makes the heart pump better.'"

"Yeah, and they do a lot of these bypasses that aren't needed," says Lear. "In some hospitals this is a rip-off for a big fee."

"Now, Lear, you are too hard on doctors and hospitals," says Rodney.

"I've read it. I'll get ten second opinions before I'll let them cut me open."

"Well, Lear," says Murphy, "the NIH booklet reports they have demonstrated 'that the great majority of patients with stable and mild or moderate symptoms can defer having a bypass operation without fear of premature death.'"

"I knew it," says Lear.

"Here they did a study with some getting surgery and others getting medicines. However, where there was substantial narrowing in all three vessels, the surgery best served the patients."

"I hope I don't have to make that decision." says Victor.

"Right on," says Zaroom.

"Okay, fellows, one more thing on treatment. The bypass operation has saved a lot of lives and spared a lot of pain, but NIH has been determined to find better treatments.

"One is the use of a balloon catheter. A tube with a little sausage-shaped balloon on the end is run up to the heart area through an artery, and when it reaches the blocked area the balloon is inflated to press the blockage and open the blood vessel. The doctors can watch through their equipment."

"That's so simple. Will it replace surgery?"

"They are working on it, I take it. Sounds very promising.

"Also, there are other methods being examined by NIH and NIH grantees. There is a lot of heart research going on around the country."

"What is angina?" Victor asks. "Postmaster Britt had this for a long time before he died of a heart attack."

"That is mild blockage and angina pain is less severe than other heart problems, and after it has been diagnosed, the doctor will recommend that you rest and when there is pain take a nitroglycerin tablet, which relaxes the blood vessels, or some other of a number of available drugs, and maybe there are some remedial steps the doctor will recommend."

"What else other than clogged up blood vessels causes heart attacks?" asks Victor.

"Family history, genes, but you have probably already out-grown that risk.

"We know smoking greatly increases risk, and so does obesity and a lack of exercise. Heart disease is prompted by diabetes, but diabetics have other problems. Stress and high blood pressure are causes and warnings. Some have suggested that 'Type A' behavior or personality makes you more susceptible to heart attacks.

"But to get back to Roddy's question, how do we keep from having an endangered heart?"

"Aging a cause?"

"No, it's not likely that age is a cause, but the risk of heart problems increases with age. Age brings with it an accumulation of sloppy habits on top of a more sedentary life."

Victor Beane asks, "Now, are you going to give us some things we need to do to ward off heart trouble?"

"Get rid of sloppy habits and don't get sedentary!" Joe interjects.

"Fair enough. I believe I gave you several ways to minimize cancer risk," Henry continues. "For the heart, let me just give you four. As Roddy said, the precautions are going to be about the same for each disease. But we know we should eat right--fewer fats, more fiber, reduce cholesterol--we should not smoke, and should exercise regularly, keeping weight under control and practice early detection."

" I don't believe we need to wait," says Roddy. Why don't you go ahead and list the main things we need to do to cut the risks of cancer, cardiovascular, and most of the others."

"Sure. Let's try, and we will add more if we come across additional precautions for other diseases."

"I have been jotting down the various pieces of advice," Henry says, "and here is what I come up with. Remember, not only precautions against the development of diseases, but to delay the aging process, protect the vital organs.

"First, the negatives. Nobody denies the effect of smoking on cancer and cardiovascular disease, so quit. Limit the amount of alcohol.

"Second, exercise. Keep fit. Lose fat. Exercise muscles. Keep moving.

"Third, eat right--avoid cholesterol and fats, salt if that applies to you, get roughage and a balanced diet and adequate nutrients.

"Finally, conduct self-examination for cancer signs, heart pains, and any irregularities, and get regular health check-ups, and don't put off or fudge on required treatment."

"Well that ain't too complicated," says Lear. "Four things."

"Sure, we can handle that. Let's tag them 'The Final Four,'" says Joe Zaroom.

"That's a good basketball term," says Will, "but how about calling it the first four, or the foremost four?"

"Or the fearsome four," says Roddy.

"Hold on, what if Henry finds more than four?"

"We'll think of another tag," says Joe Zaroom.

"Meanwhile, its the Final Four to dodge the diseases and slow old man aging. Good going, Henry!"

"We ought to be able to handle--to remember--four things."

"Well one of your good health rules is to keep moving. So we need to move on, Henry," says Roddy. "I've got a man at the office who wants to give me some money."

"Fair enough," says Henry. "I wish I did. See you fellows on Friday. I still have some chronic diseases for us to out-fox."

"See you next Friday."

Chapter Five

HIGH BLOOD AND AVOIDING STROKE

*T*he group was already in place when Victor Beane, the last to arrive, hurries to the table.

"Violet, don't forget me."

"Never do that, Mr. Beane. You want your prunes?"

"Why not?"

"I've got all the orders, says Violet. "Start the class, professor."

Victor Beane takes his seat, talking. "Henry, what do you find about cholesterol? Some say it doesn't matter. Then there is good cholesterol and bad cholesterol. And advertisements tell us something will reduce cholesterol, and it turns out to be insignificant. And other food boxes proclaim 'No Cholesterol' when there never was any cholesterol in that kind of food. Is the public getting a snow job about cholesterol?"

"Maybe, but most experts think cholesterol is a prominent villain in heart disease. Some think otherwise. In clogged vessels, it's there, but is it the cause? I think the medical world has much more to learn about cholesterol.

"I have this *Nutrition Action Newsletter*, June 1989, that tells us it is impossible to predict how much a food will raise or lower your cholesterol from where it is now. That's because so much depends on your genes and on what you currently eat. Some say it's the excess cholesterol made by the liver that is the villain. I'll get some more information about cholesterol."

"So, move it on Professor," calls out Joe Zaroom, "What's next?"

"Well why don't I hit you with stroke, Joe? Here the blood flow to the brain is interrupted. Same as loss of oxygen and nutrients will kill heart muscle, so will it kill brain cells. I have some material from the National Institutes of Health.

"Stroke is the third leading cause of death. It also cripples a lot of people and puts them in nursing homes."

"The blood flow interrupted? How?"

"The most prevalent is thrombotic. You know that word. Fatty deposits, plaques you remember, can clog vessels and cut the blood supply--oxygen and nutrients--to the brain. Then there is an embolic stroke, when a clot or plaque debris from anywhere in the body breaks loose and travels to the brain where it blocks the flow of blood.

"There is another and I'd say generally worse stroke. This is called a hemorrhagic stroke. This means that a blood vessel in the brain has burst--a cerebral hemorrhage. About a third of the strokes are this kind."

"What causes the hemorrhage?"

"Mostly by what is called an aneurysm, a blood vessel pops. It might be that it was flawed from birth. It might be a result of continued high blood pressure--hypertension--which has created little blisters or weak spots. It can also be a second step of the strokes I've mentioned--where cells are already killed due to loss of blood supply."

"Frightening, Henry. Now, what happens when you have a stroke?"

"Simply put, part of your brain is incapacitated.

"Depending on what part of the brain is damaged, the impairment may be of speech, memory, thinking and comprehension, and the use and control of muscles, including vision. Your limbs can be paralyzed, and you might know what you want to say and can't find the word, or find the words and they make no sense, or not be able to talk at all. It is possible that there is no muscular damage, just damage to the ability to verbalize your thoughts."

"I remember Alexander Whitmore," says Roddy. "After he had his stroke and could get around, had plenty of money and would meet with a lot of people in civic projects. He always had two young secretaries with him, and they would quietly suggest the right word when he hesitated. But he was sharp as a tack. Knew what he was doing. Just couldn't come up with the right word."

"It's bad stuff. And usually one side of the body. That right?" Beane asks.

"Because of the way the brain is constructed and how it relates to the body. As you might guess, right side damage impairs the left side of the body and vice versa. Also, left side damage might affect speech and language."

"And some strokes are much worse than others," adds Will Mack. "Look at Billy McArthur, had a stroke, and back to playing tennis in two months. And poor old Vestal can't move without a nurse and walker."

"That's right," reports Joe Zaroom, "Vestal's wife told me he had a hemorrhage, an artery exploded she said."

"An aneurysm. That's the way it happens," says Henry. "The artery has a weakened area wall at some spot, and it suddenly blows out like an intertube.

"Then there can be a stroke much less severe than Billy had," Henry continues. "It is a transient attack--called, let me see, a TIA, transient ischemic attack, and all of us better watch out for these. It is a temporary and brief interruption, maybe a temporary speech, visual, or movement impairment, or dizziness. You need to see the doctor. This is the prediction of a possible stroke. See your doctor right away."

"And what can the doctor do?"

"He can tell you that a TIA is a warning sign that might predict a real stroke. See the doctor!"

"You are right," says Will Mack. "Strokes, or some of them, can be prevented by drugs, if you start soon enough. My doctor prescribed an aspirin a day after I had a numb left hand. Said it would reduce the likelihood of a stroke."

"Maybe," Henry answers, "but ask your doctor. There are stronger medicines. But let your doctor tell you. I'm not practicing medicine. Aspirin does indeed tend to thin the blood. And in some situations, surgery is needed to remove clots, but this is a chancy proposition."

"And," says Lear, "some people can't take aspirin."

"I don't doubt that. See your doctor."

"You got to catch it soon enough, that's the key," says Lear. "You remember Marida Turlington, our secretary at the shop. Been there since Adam and Eve. She got flushed and faint and the girls took her out to the hospital and Doc Bershoc called and said it was serious, that he thought she was going to have a stroke. I said, 'Hell, Doc, gonna have--don't let her have it, you got her there with all that hospital equipment.' He said they didn't know how to stop it. Sure enough about ten that night she had it. I reckon maybe they kept it from being as bad. She's still limping and smiling, as she says."

"Good point Lear."

Murphy goes on, "After a stroke, physical therapy is needed. It sometimes can be long and difficult. But it can be successful."

"Now, Henry, get to the nut in the peanut," Joe Zaroom says. "What causes strokes? What do we do to keep them from happening?"

"That's the next logical question, Joe. High on the villains' list is atherosclerosis. Certainly what is done to avoid the buildup of plaque--the defenses against heart attack apply here, 'The Final Four.'

"Also, a stroke can be caused by some diseases--sickle cell, heart disease, excessive red cell count, and especially diabetes. Those are things your doctor will have to care for, and they cause only a small percentage of strokes.

"High blood pressure, however, is the number-one stroke villain."

"Okay, tell us about high blood pressure," says Zaroom.

"I've got the government booklet right here--all marked up. Blood pressure is the force against the walls of the arteries. When the heart beats, the pressure is normally about 120. Between beats, it should be about 80. If it gets above 140 and 90, that is defined as hypertension or high blood pressure."

"Hypertension means, does it, that we are super tense and that increases the blood pressure?" asks Joe Zaroom.

"Not at all. It is a medical term for high blood pressure. It can occur in relaxed, calm people."

"I can grasp that, but what causes high blood pressure--or hypertension?"

"Medical science doesn't really know. There is a guess that it's a genetic condition, so in time we will know. For the present, the best I can determine, there are two main conditions that cause high blood pressure--salt accumulation in the body that causes the heart to pump harder, which increases the blood pressure.

"Second, the tiny blood vessels that constrict when the adrenaline flows, which is the way we get tensed up for danger or challenge, don't work right. They stay tensed up when you don't need them. And by definition that is hypertension--and it can have dangerous consequences.

"Let me add that sometimes a disease causes these arteries to constrict, but that is a puzzle yet to be solved."

"But professor, how do you know you got it?"

"Let me quote NIH. 'High blood pressure has no symptoms, so a person is not able to tell. . . .' How do you know you have high blood pressure? Only by having your blood pressure tested. You have all had the sleeve wrapped around your arm while the nurse listens with a stethoscope. They find the numbers I was talking about. The nurse tells you whether it is not normal. And then you need medical advice as to what to do."

"What to do?" asks Vic Beane.

"Depends on how severe your condition. Your doctor has to answer that question of what to do."

"I mean what to do to keep your blood pressure normal?"

"Maybe you can't. Let me refer to the NIH booklet. We are told exercise and loss of weight are good for us, smoking and excessive alcohol are bad for blood pressure, reducing tension is advisable, salt is bad for some people, but--and it is a big but--let me quote: 'As you can see, cutting out smoking, losing weight, exercising, relaxing more, and most especially, reducing your salt and fatty food intake, are all very good for you. But except in less severe cases, none of these will by itself effectively lower elevated blood pressure over time. To achieve this, in most cases, you must use certain medications and usually continue to take them indefinitely.'"

"That's bad news, I'd say."

"Sure, the medicine controls but does not cure, but the good news is that the medicine works and you can go on with your life and work in every normal way."

"Trouble with medication is the side effects" says Victor. "Scotty Carr almost developed palsy before they took him off of the medicine. True?"

"It wouldn't be good to generalize from that. Drugs may be necessary, and many are available, and new medicines are being developed. The answer is to rely on your doctor, if you need medicine. Then, you, with his advice, watch for side effects."

"So, Professor, sum it up," says Joe Zaroom.

"Final Four. Smoking and excessive use of alcohol should be avoided. Final Four. Exercise. Final Four. Watch your diet, especially salt, especially your weight. Final Four. Get your blood pressure tested. If it is high, follow your doctor's advice on stress management."

"Why avoid salt?"

"Probably not necessary if you don't have a blood pressure problem. It is a matter of salt not being properly eliminated, and I haven't found a good answer as to why it works as it does."

"I've got two questions, professor," says Victor. "Does stress cause strokes?"

"My government book says no, not directly, but remember stress is associated with heart disease, as is high blood pressure and Type A personalities. And heart disease relates to strokes. So excessive stress is not something to be disregarded as age makes you more likely to suffer a stroke."

"Well what is stress?"

"Ah, not easily defined. Rather, the word is used to describe the personal conflict with an environment, and the coping. How does one adjust to the maladjustment that is stress? Here we are.

"Erdman B. Palmore of Duke studied five major life events-- retirement, spouse's retirement, major medical events, widowhood and departure of the last child from home, and concluded that it was the frail or at risk older person who needed professional help in coping--rather than the average elder. It appears that many of these potentially stressful events are less serious for those with good physical, psychological, and social resources.

"And what is your second question?"

"Oh, yes. How do you know you might have an aneurysm? Is there any way to tell?"

"Not easily. A sudden severe headache at the base of your head may be the first sign. In the neck artery there may be a pulsating, swishing sound you can detect. Usually, it slips up on you, so see your doctor if you note any signs.

"One final thing. Strokes are debilitating, but recovery is the pattern. There is much known about therapy for recovery."

"Wait a minute, Henry. What good is therapy if you die. Doesn't a stroke generally kill you?"

"Well, Roddy, over a third do die, according to the book. But those who don't can get treatment and can get better. It takes spunk and determination sometimes. It's easier for some than others. And, I suppose it is both true and sad that sometimes the damage is just too severe for much repair."

"Tell us about the ones spunk and determination can cure."

"Cure may not be the word, but successful treatment and recovery are possible. Here is what NIH tells us. Treatment starts the moment the doctor sees the patient. So don't delay if you begin to have symptoms.

"Let's go back a step. The brain, or parts of it, which fail to get the oxygen and nutrients, struggle to compensate, and when it can hold on no longer, the brain fails and the stroke occurs, and the damage spreads as time passes. The urgent task is to stop the spread. A PET scanner, and other technologies, help see the damaged, the dead and surrounding threatened areas, and guides the doctors in stopping and reversing, if possible, the damage.

"Let me quote the NIH booklet: 'When a stroke occurs, the clock starts running and patients must obtain medical help promptly or risk losing vital brain function.'"

"And Henry, I suppose, there is much going on in research."

"Certainly. Let me quote again. 'Today, we are learning that there are many ways to treat stroke, both independently and in combination with a variety of therapies.'"

"Getting back to what we can do," asks Victor, "is there anything other than our magic four steps?"

"Yes, a funny addendum. I have read several places that the chance of a stroke is increased by a beer belly, or a pot and a spare tire, or as more sedately, and authoritatively, put by the NIH, 'abdominal obesity.' It is not just fat, but fat in that place. So start your sit-ups."

"And watch your diet."

"Now, Henry, can you tell us about rehabilitation?"

"That's beyond my scope. My assignment is old age and how to get through it in good health.

"I can tell you rehabilitation for strokes is possible in many--in most--cases, but that is for the doctors to prescribe when you get there--which I hope you don't."

"And that is about it," says Rodney. "I've got to go. See you--when? Next Tuesday."

"No, two weeks from Tuesday," says Lear. "Joe and I are going fishing."

"Right. I forgot."

Roddy is already on his feet and Henry stands up, "I suppose I'll see you when I see you. Have a good time!"

Chapter Six

SEX, WRINKLES, AND ARTHRITIS

For two weeks the big table at Gus's stayed empty at breakfast. Now Lear and Joe Zaroom have returned from their annual fishing trip. Victor Beane's visiting ninety-year-old aunt and her new husband have gone home. Henry's announced sabbatical is over.

It is a July morning, the early sun is in the sky, and Henry Murphy is swinging along Freedom Street, talking to himself. *Old Harry Truman didn't just walk every morning, he walked briskly, on parade. He walked at the pace World War One soldiers marched. Would remind people that he was taking 120 steps a minute. I'm not walking, I'm not meandering, I'm not strolling--I'm marching downtown. Shoulders back. Hup, two, three, four . . ."*

He waves at a passing car, the driver having tapped the horn. *Old man Macintosh, going out to look at his crops. Bet they need rain.*

Henry pushes the door open, glances to the rear of the restaurant, and stops before Gus. "Anybody here?" he asks.

"Me," says Gus, "and by the way, good morning."

"Oh, good morning, Gus. Glad to see you. Are you doing all right?"

"Same as always. But Violet has missed you."

"Well, I'm glad to see you, Gus. I reckon most of the boys will be along."

"I hope so. Go on back and get some coffee."

Henry moves to the rear, to his table, and Violet meets him with a cup of coffee.

"I'm sure glad to see you. It's like being unemployed when you guys are not here--not that I make any money off you," Violet laughed. "I told my mama you were all Depression tippers."

"Now Violet, I'm so glad to see you. You brighten my day. You start it off with your wonderful smile."

"Thank you, Mr. Henry. You want to wait to order?"

"I think I'll wait, Violet." Henry sits at his place.

"Mr. Henry, let me ask you something. All this talk about old age, and sickness. Do you think you can hold back time? I don't like to hear about it. It's sad."

"Well, Violet, we seem to be enjoying it. Maybe it gives us something to cling to, something to want. When you are younger you have goals and ambitions and are striving to achieve something, to get from here to there. Then that all becomes the past. In perspective, not much is urgent, maybe not very important. Lear Jones can no longer hope to become the manager of the company. Mr. Beane can no longer dream of leaving the post office to make a million dollars. I will never be a distinguished professor. Will Mack probably never wanted to do anything but run a school, but all of that is now behind him. Roddy Thomas is coasting on something good that he built. Joe is through selling cheap shoes and suits and is back to his first love, baseball. It seems to me, Violet, that too many people at this time of their lives simply let go. Now, we are saying there is another adventure. Does that make any sense? People can live many more years in good health, enjoying their families and friends, doing some good in the neighborhood and community, free of the old stress and strain of the ambitions of the young. But to get rid of the stress doesn't mean you let go of the plank that has kept you floating in this vast ocean called life. You'd sink and drown. We are talking about catching another plank. It will be fun to beat the odds. It adds purpose to life. I get a new charge out of knowing I can most likely do it. I'm holding to a new plank. Does that make any sense, Violet?"

Lear Jones and Rodney have come in together, and Bob Beane is walking toward the rear. They all greet as if they had not seen each other for years. Joe Zaroom immediately arrives and slaps all on their shoulders. They all shuffle around and sit down, and Violet stands there with her order pad.

"What'll it be, gents?"

Lear Jones is the first to speak.

"You got any cereal? Corn flakes? What kinds of cereals are there other than corn flakes?"

"We got corn flakes. And about everything else. There are more kinds of cereals than there are sparrows."

"I'll take the corn flakes and fruit and skim milk. You got strawberries?"

"No, but I'll bring you some fresh blueberries."

Rodney had followed this exchange very carefully. "Damn, Lear old boy, it's a jolt to see a great institution crumble right in front of you. You're the cholesterol king. Fried eggs, sausage, and hash brown potatoes, toast and butter. Say it ain't so!"

"You turkeys never have had any will power." Lear was grinning. "I listened to Henry. My blood pressure is too high. My mother and grandmother did die from cancer. My daddy died with a heart attack. Do you think I've been listening to Henry like it was the Cosby TV show? I heard what he said. The difference is I've got will power."

"Marvelous to behold," says Beane. "Bring me the same, Violet."

"Don't all of you do this," says Violet. "You're going to make me cry."

"Don't cry, Violet. Bring me the pancakes and crisp bacon," says Rodney.

Henry orders dry whole wheat toast. "Maybe all this study will serve a good purpose, after all."

"The hell you say," smiles Will Mack. "You have succeeded in ruining the best meal of the day. And now that you've got Lear on pig feed, what are you going to do about his smoking?"

"I won't ask," says Henry, with a satisfied expression. "I've got a dozen more ailments to talk about."

"Let me tell you about the fish we caught," Joe exclaims. "Me and Lear set all the new records!"

"Don't tell us," drawls Victor, "and I won't tell you about Aunt Matilda's new husband."

Joe tells anyhow, and Lear joins in. In time, Violet picks up the used dishes.

"Henry," says Roddy, with a mischievous grin, "I know you don't like to talk about sex, so I am going to quote what the National Institute on Aging presented, compiled by Mryna Lewis: 'One question that is often asked is, "Do *all* older people want an active sex life?"'

"Where did you get that paper?" Henry demands almost.

"I'm a researcher, too. I got Charlie to put me on the mailing list for *Age Page*. What's a Congressman for if not to send free publications?"

"Well," Henry is slightly huffy. "I'm glad you did. All of you should be bringing in materials. Whatever you run across. What's the answer, Roddy?"

"The answer, of course, is 'no.' Here's what she wrote. 'Some people never have been interested in sexual activity. Others have lost interest somewhere along the way and have no desire to recapture it. Still others have made the deliberate decision to share sex with one specific partner and when illness or death intervenes, sexual activity ends.'"

Roddy looked around. "Shall I go on?"

"Sure."

"Talk," says Zaroom.

"'It is important to recognize and respect each individual's personal choice.' I'm reading the report. 'Today, many older people want--and are able to lead--an active, satisfying sex life. Sometimes, however, physical or emotional problems affect sexual expression. . . . In general, women experience little serious loss of sexual capacity due to age alone. . . . For many older women, sexual activity is determined by the age and health of their partner. . . . Older men often notice more distinct changes in sexual functioning than women, although these changes vary greatly from man to man. . . . However, these changes do not mean that a man is becoming impotent.'

"This is straight from the National Institute on Aging. 'If a man is in reasonably good health and if he has had a fulfilling sex life, he will probably continue to function sexually throughout the rest of his life, unless illness stops him.'

"Let me read some quotes: 'Men's interest in sex appears to decline little with age. . . . Prescription drugs are believed to be responsible for about 25 percent of male impotence. . . . Most drug-related sexual problems are probably caused by alcohol abuse.'

"Then she philosophizes. There are 'two languages of sex,' she says. 'The first is typical of the young. . . . The second is typical of the older individuals--it is learned rather than instinctive, and it is more mature emotionally, as well as physically. Indeed there is sex after 60. As men and women age, they continue to express their sexuality and their need for human warmth and companionship.' There's my homework, professor."

"Well, I thank you for that" says Henry. "It sure is good to have a resident sex specialist."

Will Mack speaks. "That research lady Roddy read from has stated the matter too pat. It is appropriate to redefine the definition of sex, giving its full meaning of tenderness and caring and loving concern that goes on all day and night, and all of that is quite enough at my age.

"The word is limited too often to one quick act. It is the quiet touch, the loving pat, that gets more and more important. There are mountains and valleys in sex life, starting out fiery and then, funny thing, the product of sex can destroy the joy of sex. Children! They have problems, or we think they do, that overshadow the free caring and companionship of newlyweds.

"There was a brash right-wing senator some years ago who tried to make a big name for himself by legislating at every turn against abortion, holding hearings, and his *coup de grace* was, 'Ah, but doctor, when does life begin?' He would then make his stump speech for voter consumption when the doctor didn't give him the answer he wanted. One old constituent got fed up with the senator's antics, and wrote a letter to the editor saying, 'I can tell old Jack when life begins: *When the children leave home and the dog dies!*'

"Then you can be newlyweds again if you haven't forgotten how. No more going to bed to bicker about the children's' daily dash for hellfire. No more arguing about Susie's party dress or Junior's getting into the wine . . . time to be newlyweds again. Trouble is the paint has peeled, the clock has rusted, so you have to work at it. And it is worth it. And as you get older the shared burdens and ordeals endured tend to bring you closer together, if you don't fight it."

Murphy picks up, "I had the notes from wise and reliable Alex Comfort, before I got these two great volunteers, who wrote, 'Sexual requirement and sexual capacity are lifelong. Even if and when actual intercourse is impaired by infirmity, other sexual needs persist, including closeness. . . being valued as a man or a woman.'

"You people keep changing the subject. That wasn't in my lesson plan. Now that we've talked about pleasures of old age, let's talk about some ailments of old age. I'll come back to chronic diseases."

"Speaking of ailments, look at that."

Lear sticks out his hand between Beane and Henry Murphy, and says, "Look at that. An old man's hand. What about all those brown splotches?"

"That's not in my lesson plan either, but let me shuffle through these papers. I've got something. Here it is. Dr. Albert Klingman of Penn. Wrote that the skin's 'primary function . . . [is to] protect the body from . . . insults.'"

"Sounds reasonable," says Roddy. "Good to have protection. That includes insults from Zaroom?"

"O.K.," Henry goes on, "if you are so smart. Dr. Klingman says, 'No one ever dies of skin failure,' that the skin can 'carry out it's protective function adequately throughout life.'

"It is true, and I'm summarizing, the skin might get a little wrinkled, dry, loose, sometimes itchy, after 70, and less natural oil secretes, and sweating decreases, but all of that can be handled."

"A little palm in the palm," interjects Vic Beane. "Or Intensive Care or Ponds, or something similar, and I am free to admit, every morning I grease up my legs, arms, hands, and face."

"No wonder I can't see any wrinkles on you," said Will Mack, "and all the time I thought it was just that your skin was stretched so tight over your fat layer."

"I can read it right here," says Henry. "The good doctor writes, 'Everyone over 65 should use a moisturizer every day, especially on dry areas of skin.'

"Does he say anything about a face lift for wrinkles?" Rodney asks.

"Oh, yes," Henry responds, "He seems to approve completely cosmetic surgery for sags and wrinkles, facial blotches and spots, including chemical peel for new and fresh skin, but none of you has got the guts to go to a plastic surgeon."

"Not for me," Roddy laughs. "For you know who. She's been talking about a face lift for years. I'm all for it."

"Let me have the last word," Henry says. "The doctor says that 'most geriatricians do not consider this subject very important because no one dies of old skin. . . . But as the skin grows older . . . doesn't look good . . . can make people miserable. For these reasons, the problems of aging skin are very serious. . . to some people.'"

"Not to me, it ain't," says Joe. "If it will hold me together like a plastic grocery bag, I'm satisfied. But what about skin cancer? Can't that kill you?"

"I suppose the doctor didn't blame that on the skin," Henry answered. "We've talked about it. Not too much sun, and examine yourself for moles and growths.

"Now, I've got time to talk about one other thing. What will it be? Chronic illness? I've covered cancer and cardiovascular, the two big killers. I've talked about strokes. I've mentioned a half-dozen others."

"You didn't answer my question about the splotches on my hands," says Lear.

"Gosh, I didn't. You are sharp, Lear. Don't let me change the subject on you. But I don't have the answer. I'll look for something."

"Can we talk about the disabilities of old age?" asks Roddy. "There are killers and there are things you wish would kill you-- shingles."

"Sure. Debilitating diseases that mostly hit older people. Let's start with arthritis."

"I already have," says Lear.

"You are in good company. More people suffer from arthritis than any other impediment. It affects the joints and connective tissues, fingers, knees, hips, and the spine, could attack almost any joints. It hurts because inflamed joints rub against each other, or little bone or calcium growths might cause discomfort and pain, or might pinch a nerve, which will spread the pain."

"Rheumatism," Bob Beane calls out. "Rheumatiz. One thing that I remember about my granddaddy was that he would stand up and groan, 'The old rheumatiz has got me.'"

"There are two chief kinds of arthritis--osteoarthritis and rheumatoid arthritis. Which sounds worse, Joe?"

"What? Oh, oleo sounds worse."

"Osteo--and that is the least serious. Osteoarthritis is what might slap all of us to some degree.

"Tell," says Joe.

"They say osteoarthritis probably can't be avoided, and can't be cured. Doctors can prescribe non-steroidal anti-inflammatory drugs, the doctor might just prescribe aspirin or some pain killer. The point of the medicine is to reduce inflammation as well as pain. Sometimes a heating pad or hot bath can help."

"You read about the arthroscope on the sports pages," interjects Joe Zaroom.

"Can't that help?"

"Surgeons can remove little growths, or cartilage or other tissue, and that operation is simplified with the arthroscope. They can also correct arthritis by replacing hips, knees, and now just about any joint. But you don't want that kind of operation at the first sign of pain."

"But Henry, remember our main question. How do we avoid arthritis?" asks Lear Jones.

"I didn't find any satisfactory answer. Some say susceptibility is quite likely inherited. I didn't find any satisfactory explanation of cause. Another guess is that it comes from inaction that advancing age promotes, but that doesn't add up, it seems to me. It could be an accumulation of little bumps, strains, and bruises. It can also come from too much exercise and from injuries. It also, say in the spine, hips, and knees, could be caused by being too fat."

"Okay, what can we do?"

"I've always thought it was aggravated, if not caused by stress and worry and distress, but I can't prove that," says Will Mack.

"I haven't come across such a reference."

"I can cite a lot of examples."

"I don't doubt it, and stress causes other disabilities, but science doesn't know--yet. Right now we can guess at ways to avoid or relieve osteoarthritis. I take it that there are three things.

"First, regular exercise of joints and muscles is a preventative step. We are going to devote a whole breakfast to exercise, but it may be an important way to ward off arthritis. How many of you exercise your fingers regularly?"

Roddy laughs. "Joe is always pointing fingers."

"Fair enough. But here is a serious point: If you already have arthritic joints, rest helps, and exercise helps. Don't overdo either. Don't neglect either. The joints will hurt most when not used for a long period, or when used too strenuously for too long."

"And," says Will Mack, "may I add, don't fret and worry, cast off your cares, try to overcome stress and distress. I believe there is a connection."

"Sounds reasonable. Good advice in any event. I have seen some hints that adequate vitamin C might be a deterrent. This is one more reason to get enough vitamin C.

"What causes it? There are a hundred different conditions of osteoarthritis, many symptoms, many causes. There is a fair amount of research going on."

"There must be a common cause somewhere," says Will Mack.

"Aren't we making arthritis sound too simple?" asks Will Mack. "I know some people who suffer tremendously, whose hands are almost useless, who can't open a child-safe medicine bottle, who have a hard time turning the key to the front door."

"I don't mean to do that," Henry answers. "Sol Thacker can't get a good night's sleep for pain in his hands and wrists. I don't discount it at all. Forty million Americans have arthritis in their hands or feet. It is a damnable disease. It is said that everyone over seventy has some form of degenerative joint disease."

"Tell about rheumatoid arthritis" says Victor.

"That is the more serious, and less common, arthritis. Almost all the joints can be affected, sometimes all at once, and the joints become swollen, and very painful. They will be reddened and hot. This disease also can affect lungs, spleen, and maybe your heart. It can be controlled, but it causes deformities. I will just mention it, because it is not an old-age disease as much as a middle-age. It is likely to be hereditary, a matter of genes. If you have escaped it in middle age, the odds are in your favor."

"What about osteoporosis? Is that related?" asks Victor.

"Related, but something else. It relates to the bones. That's what osteo means, and it is a debilitating disease that in some degree affects three-fourths of older women. It is certainly one of our bad chronic diseases.

"It causes weakened bones, and results in fractures--chiefly hips, and forearms and vertebrae. It has to do with a loss of estrogen and inadequate calcium. Calcium from 1000 to 2500 milligrams a day is the safe treatment. Calcium carbonate is the recommended and cheapest form of supplemental calcium. I got that from a big book named *Diet and Health*, which I'm going to talk about later."

"It also causes its victims to be stooped?" asks Victor.

"That's it. And it probably can be halted in some cases, but it has not been possible to restore loss of the inner bone. There is research to build back inner bone structure by controlled exercise. That is in the future."

"Gosh, time is flying," says Roddy. "I've got to go."

"It's next Friday, is it?" says Henry. "I want to talk about the process of aging, how we might understand it and slow the process. It is a fascinating topic."

"You mean what is aging?"

"That's right."

"Sounds great."

Chapter Seven

CORRALLING FREE RADICALS

Joe and Henry have arrived and are talking to Lear when Rodney comes in and sits down to the cup of coffee Violet brings him.

"You know," says Roddy, "When I woke up this morning, the clock seemed to be running so fast. I sat on the edge of the bed and watched the sweep-second hand whirling around. God, time is running out. And there is so much I want to do. We are coming to the end of the line. I went to Washington when I was 15 years old and I rode the streetcar to the end of the line. I had paid a dime when I got on in the center of town. I thought I would ride back. 'All off, everybody out, end of the line!' the conductor insisted. I had another dime but I was saving that for two hot dogs. So I got off. End of the line. This is as far as she goes. And the clock is racing. The hands are twirling. I pulled the plug on the clock. The hands stopped. No. That's not the answer--that's worse! I plugged it back in.

"Well, I thought. To hell with it. Let her run. I'll run, too. I got up and did my exercises and went to the shower."

"Only way to go," says Joe.

The others arrive and Violet takes the orders. Most have finished the breakfast when Henry Murphy pulls around his chair and straddles it so he can see everybody, and takes out his little notebook.

"You've noticed I found that I couldn't just report on one book after the other. I have to read a bunch and draw on them for each subject. This is the tenth notebook I've filled," Henry thumbs it open and smiles.

"Well I met several new friends recently. They are Carl Eisdorfer, George Maddox, Franklin Williams, Richard Cutler, and a Russian named V.V. Frolkis. They gave me the baseline for the points I want to make."

"Where'd you meet 'em?" asks Joe.

"I'll have to admit I met them the same place I met Sir Walter Scott and William Shakespeare--in the library. But I'd like to meet them personally--I don't mean Shakespeare and Scott."

"You can meet a lot of smart people there," says Roddy. "Now tell us what they told you."

"Something we need to know: What is the aging process?"

"You mean," asks Will Mack, "what happens to our bodies--as distinguished from disease, our state of mind, finances, and so on-- as we grow older?"

"That's it. Not what illnesses occur, but aging, damage to our cells, our arteries and blood vessels, our vital organs, wearing out, and the whole business of DNA and the signals it, or they, give or don't give to parts of the body."

"And why these things happen faster in some people than in others?" asks Lear. "Look at Vic. The things working on me ain't been working on him. Why does he look so young?"

"Clean living," says Victor, "And Henry, our point is how to slow down the aging process?"

"Sure. That's what we are looking for," says Henry. "What are the agents that slow or speed aging? That is the second point, after we try to understand just what is the process of aging."

"Agents? Things we can take?"

"No, things in the body's system. But my third point will be what actions, positive and defensive, can we consciously take that might slow the process?"

"That would mean avoiding diseases," Will Mack continues.

"That's something else. I want to look at more of the things we can do for ourselves to slow the process of aging. Of course there is overlap. We think our Final Four will help avoid the chronic diseases, but they will also slow aging, and now we want to understand how that might be."

"Can we consciously slow the aging process?"

Henry nods. "I think we can. Let me read what V.M. Dil'man wrote. 'We use life's blessings every day. We age as the days pass, therefore we must counteract aging daily.'"

"So how do we counteract aging?" asks Will Mack.

"Ah. That is our main point. We don't get to the end of the life span just because we avoid the chronic diseases," says Henry. "There is another hurdle. The aging process can be running like Roddy's clock. We need to slow it down."

"That's our question. How can the aging process be slowed?" says Roddy, "Whatever it is."

"Let's look at that step by step. We already know the control of dread childhood diseases, the new drugs that control infectious diseases, get more people to and beyond the former life expectancy.

"We understand that, but don't miss the point: Can we slow down--stretch out--the aging process?"

"Henry, let me interrupt, please," says Rodney. "I have a chart here that clarified longevity for me. Of course age 70-plus--life expectancy--is an average, and we all want to live beyond that--some of us have already. It is not that 70 is *the* age, 70 plus is the average--half the people will reach that age--and there is no suggestion that 70 is an ideal age to reach, or is about where we have to check out."

"You've got it right."

"Listen to this: 'Statistically, we can expect to live longer the older we get. This chart shows that when you are 70 you have a life expectancy of 11 years. At 80, you get a new lease, you have a life expectancy of 7 more years. At 90, the life expectancy, statistically, is 3.8 years. And remember that "life expectancy" is the *average*, not the top limit.

"Now the renewable leases get shorter. At 95, half will make it to 98, and the others who make it to 100, will be spotted two and one-half more years, and remember that is the average. You might do better, and if you reach 110 then your life expectancy, the average, is a year and a half.'"

"So hang in there, baby!" exclaimed Joe Zaroom. "Wow--110! That's the average so we can go beyond, Professor Murphy. Right?"

"A little bit, I reckon, Joe, but don't get carried away. A lot more than statistics made it possible for those people to reach the upper upper brackets."

"But that's not the whole story," says Will Mack. "We live longer because disease is conquered or delayed by lifestyle and luck. But aging goes on. Why?"

"Let me read you what Dr. George Maddox wrote: He notes, as we have already learned, longer life 'will depend on control of specific diseases. . . .' Of greater importance, he says, is the 'control of the intrinsic physiological processes of the human body.' That is to say, 'the aging and death of human cells. . . .' If scientists can get a handle on that, Dr. Maddox says, 'a life expectancy of 100 years is possible, some scientists maintain.' Expectancy, not life span, he said."

"That means the aging process can't be stopped, but can be slowed?"

"Yes, we hope," says Henry, "so let me go back to the first point of this discussion: What is aging?

"I have already referred to Dr. Carl Eisdorfer, a pioneer in the modern study of gerontology. Let me summarize his hypothesis about the theory of aging.

"Eisdorfer wrote that the process of aging 'involves the death of cells.' This is so 'because the cell fails to reproduce itself accurately,' and 'most cells in the body must be reproduced at a fairly regular rate.'"

"Do we know why the cells fail to reproduce?" asks Will Mack.

"That's the puzzle. The child grows quickly as cells reproduce rapidly. The rate of reproduction slows down, on schedule, as scheduled, as we mature and grow older. This is normal, and it apparently is the DNA system that programs the required stabilization as the child becomes an adult.

"Into the adult years, constant cell replication occurs and then, as we age, the production of new cells slows and then virtually stops. The 'renovation' of the cells comes to an end and the vital organs are about 'worn out.'"

"So, Doc," says Will Mack, "back to my question. What causes cells to lose their zip and fail to replicate themselves?"

""Richard G. Cutler, in a book edited by Alelman and Roth, tells a fascinating example, relevant to the aging of humans, the 'instant aging' of the octopus, which ages out and dies as soon as it reproduces. It is programmed that way genetically. The same is true of the Pacific coast salmon. All animals seem to be genetically programmed to age out--humans at about 100 years?

"So we are programmed. Can we change the program," insists Will Mack.

"You understand," says Henry, "a hypothesis is not a fact. Let me see if I can explain what I read from Dr. Cutler. One thought is that a distinct set of genes are there to prolong life by protecting and repairing the bodily functions."

"The immune system?"

"Something much broader. Our immune system fights invaders. These are genes that, among other things, might repair the DNA damage, or see to it that the damage is repaired."

"Now, don't take me too fast," says Joe.

"Okay, let me give you Dr. Cutler's analogy. Some scientists believe that we age like an automobile where all parts are designed to last about the same, and if you are going to make that car last longer you must improve all parts--in human longevity terms an almost impossible job.

"The hypothesis Cutler suggests is that you don't have to build better parts, you just need one of these computerized machines that roams around and repairs or directs the repair of any one part of the automobile that is weakened or damaged. In the body the job is done by the longevity determinant genes--LDGs."

"That is the theory--not the fact?" asks Joe.

"Sure, sure, but let me tell you how they got there. The best I can do is in simple terms. If you want to know more, read the book and the many more that he footnotes."

"Your body, Joe, we are just now understanding, is a package of information--information on how your cells are to be replicated, for one thing. The key to long life is that information package. Your reach toward maximum life span is determined by how long that information is kept correct and not garbled.

"Dr. Cutler goes on to explain that to extend life it is necessary to extend the life span of the 'sets of information.' Find a way to prolong the vitality of the information sets, find a way to protect, repair or replace the information sets, and then the life span will be lengthened."

Says Joe, "'Splain that to me."

"To understand that, we need to know that DNA--which means deoxyribonucleic acid -- is where information is stored. DNA is a tiny little twisted strand in the cell, with chemicals variously arranged, that programs, like information on a computer disk, the actions of cells and organs and body mechanisms."

"The DNA note pad or computer disk is part of the physical body, but what is written on it is not?" asks Will Mack.

"One way to put it.

"And the message attached is what keeps life going, and going properly. Rub out the message, smear it, blur it, on any little cell's note pad, and the life process is damaged to some degree."

"True."

"So," Will Mack says, "if this is a correct theory, extending healthy life is a matter of certain genes, or something else, protecting the DNA and its messages?"

"Yes, extending life to the fullness of the life span, but something still will cause the end of life."

"I understand the limit of life span is another question. Right now, how do we reach the full span?"

"Maybe genes. Maybe something else. Maybe we can do things to help the process. Let me go back to Dr. Cutler. 'From the origin of life' he writes 'the interaction of aging and anti-aging forces have prevailed.' He is talking Darwinism, from the emergence of life of the species to the individual human birth, this process of gene control has been evolving. This presents a valid query to science. Is the aging process necessary for life to exist?"

"That is to say," Will Mack asks, "the life process *is* the aging process?"

"Profound, but possible, in several ways. In human beings and all species inevitable causes of aging and death do exist. It could be genetic. Many think aging could arise from the harmful side effects of otherwise essential processes needed to maintain life. It could be both. And more.

"Another hypothesis helps explain that living is dying. An example of something essential to living is energy metabolism, the conversion--burning--oxidizing--of food, but that creates something called free radicals, which are continuously damaging cells in a process of aging, or you might say, promoting slow death."

"So what exactly are free radicals?" asks Victor.

"Good question. I'll read you a quote: 'A free radical is any chemical species with an odd number of electrons.'"

"You don't say."

"For our purposes, it is when oxygen is burning your nutrients--your food--and some oxygen molecules are left over in an unstable condition that must combine with another molecule or so, and go around looking for something else to latch on to, like a dog with a piece of bread trying to find some meat to go with it, and he might take a bite of your leg to get his meat and that damages you like a free radical damages a normal law abiding cell."

"I get the picture--I think,." Victor says.

"Let me reiterate that this is a theory. But I quote from Balin in the Adelman and Roth book: 'Free radical damage could contribute to the aging process. . . . Free radicals could cause DNA damage and mutations, which could cause, or fail to prevent, aging. To reinforce this view, let me quote Dr. John R. Johnson of Johns Hopkins in his preface to his book, *Free Radicals, Aging and Degenerative Diseases*: 'Life is a combustion process. It uses oxygen, needs oxygen, indeed its very existence depends on oxygen, and it will die for lack of oxygen perhaps more quickly than from deprivation of any other required substance. However, although oxygen is critical to life, it is also very dangerous. The danger lies in one of the possible results of chemical reactions between oxygen and other things within our environment. This one result is a substance deadly to living cells: a free radical.'

"Now, just how do free radicals take a bite out of your leg?"

"The thought is that the free radical--which physically cannot remain free--grabbing to link with other molecules does damage to the DNA, which cuts down the capacity to replicate the DNA message, or distorts the DNA message, or wipes it out."

"What has that got to do with aging?" asks Will Mack.

"Aging, according to theory you remember, embraces the inability of the cell, guided by DNA, to replicate itself."

"So, Henry, how do we defend against the free radicals? Isn't that the next question?"

"Right you are. The aging versus the anti-aging. Your system is constantly fighting off the free radicals, neutralizing them, turning them into water or something else harmless."

"So," says Will, "the time it takes to neutralize the free radicals permits damage to be done?"

"Right. The free radicals do damage by gobbling up before they can be gobbled up, and this is a big part of aging. So the key is how quickly anti-oxidants can eliminate the free radicals and thus limit the damage. So goes the theory.

"So tell us about antioxidants," says Will.

"One you need to know about is SOD, superoxide dismutase, an enzyme the body manufactures, that transforms many of the free radicals into harmless substances. (Incidentally, SOD sold by the health food people is worthless--what you need can only be manufactured in your body.)

"Other antioxidants are Vitamin E and Beta Carotene, both biological quenchers of free radicals. Vitamin C is also a free radical scavenger. So is selenium. All of the processes have not been fully explained, but this is the best information I could find."

"Back to vitamins!"

"Yes, and let me give you what I believe is Dr. Johnson's last word: 'It has not been established whether oxidative stress induced by free radical reactions and reaction products are a cause, a contributory cause, or concomitant with the aging process.'"

"But free radicals are harmful?" Victor asks.

"I believe that is a fair conclusion."

"And we fight them off with antioxidants."

"You got it. Best we know."

"Do we take antioxidants as vitamin pills?" asks Victor.

"Well, there is considerable evidence that the body manufactures antioxidants, and we ingest others, such as Beta Carotene and vitamin C, from foods we eat, such as carrots and collards. We'll talk about supplements later.

"Let me give you some more evidence from *Free Radicals, Aging, and Degenerative Diseases,* and a chapter by Denham Harmon of the University of Nebraska.

"Harmon says that 'The aging process may be the deleterious . . . changes produced by free radical reactions," so it is probable that damage--and aging--will be reduced by lowering the free radical level--by food restriction, antioxidants, and the SOD type of enzymes manufactured by our bodies."

"In line with the other fellow," says Joe.

"Sure, and Herman adds food restriction, and I take that to mean not over-eating."

"We're already trying to hold down on eating," says Rodney.

"I don't want to get too far off the subject, but in addition to the aging process, damage by free radicals may be--I say *may be*-- related to a number of diseases--cancer and cardiovascular disease, senile dementia of the Alzheimer's type, osteoarthritis, senile muscular degeneration, and Parkinson's disease."

"So they are pretty sure of the villainous nature of free radicals?" says Will Mack.

"Yes, by and large, the verdict is that free radicals are related to aging and the facilitation of some chronic diseases."

"You can see what they mean when they say living is dying. Now, can the dying part be slowed down?" asks Will Mack.

"That's our original question," says Henry. "We needed to understand the theory in order to underscore what we can do. Probably by taking in less calories, less metabolism, and a diet with all the needed anti-oxidant nutrients. Harman says the diet might include added antioxidants, Roddy, and I tend to agree. He tells us that it is reasonable to expect that such a basic diet will increase the average life expectancy . . . while possibly increasing the maximum life span slightly beyond the natural value of about 100 years.'"

"Wow," says Joe. "It is possible!"

"So why not take the pills?" says Lear.

"A good bet," says Henry. "There is still something genetic that has cut off humans, something that has defined the human life span, something that throws the master switch regardless.

"I saw in the newspaper where a scientist found a gene that deals with aging," says Roddy.

"Yes, I read that yesterday, so I went back to some books. It was Dr. Michael Rose of the University of California who had experimented with fruit flies, and Dr. Thomas Johnson of the University of Colorado who had experimented with roundworms."

"And we can be compared with worms and flies," says Joe.

"You got it, Joe boy. A gene is a gene, and now they and other researchers will look at the human genome. However, this was not an aging gene that they identified, not the genes that might be programmed to cause aging, nor genes that might retard aging. This gene didn't do either."

"So, tell," says Joe.

"Okay, our theory of free radicals is that they can be captured by scavengers and converted to something not harmful?"

"Right, by antioxidants."

"Correct. Now for the discoveries made by Dr. Rose and Dr. Johnson. Dr. Rose found the gene in fruit flies that regulates the production of SOD, so it is possible to increase SOD for an extension of life span. The gene doesn't slow aging as such, but speeds up the formation of SOD, and SOD gets rid of free radicals. Dr. Johnson manipulated the same kind of gene in roundworms and got a life extension of about 70 percent."

"So," says Will Mack, "this means that they believe that free radicals cause aging, and that the production of SOD is regulated by a gene, or genes, and if the gene can be made hyperactive, there will be produced more SOD to attack more effectively the free radicals?"

"You've got it, although the good doctors might not recognize how we are explaining it," .

"So," continues Henry, they are on to a significant discovery. As Dr. Rose reported to the American Association for the Advancement of Science, 'for the first time in human history there is a real possibility of affecting the aging process with biomedical intervention.'"

"Well, that is terrific. But what about us? We can't wait for the real possibilities. Shall we take what we can in the way of diet and supplements to do what the gene does, promote the formation of additional antioxidants?" asks Will.

"Sounds sound," says Henry.

"Yeah," says Will Mack. "If we create more antioxidants for our bodies, we do what the gene might do for the roundworms. And we know how to do that, don't we Henry?"

"Sure, sure, we think we know. But there is a lot not proven. I've already said a balanced diet helps, and Dr. Finch seems to tell us that supplements help--other writers seem to confirm this more specifically."

"So, don't take a chance, take supplements?" asks Lear.

"Well Lear, that's my opinion. Let me talk about supplements. I know Roddy is skeptical. In my view, leaving open the question of general vitamins, I think we must take anti-oxidant supplements. I believe anti-oxidants, as supplements, are extremely important to longer life--and perhaps disease prevention, and I believe the worms and the fruit flies prove we do not get enough naturally."

"Naturally?" Rodney asserts. "We can get all we need from a proper diet, and that is the word of the best doctor in town!"

"Roddy, dammit, I've never before known you to be so blind." Lear is irritated.

"What makes you smarter than Dr. Gibson?" Roddy, out of character, snarls.

"I may not be smart, but I'm not blind!" Lear yells. "Do you take the supplements, Henry?"

"Well, yes."

"How much? Give us a figure."

"I will, if you guys will calm down, but you understand it is a guess. I find no clear recommendations. Twice a day I take 500 mg of vitamin C, 50 mcg of selenium, 400 IU of vitamin E, and a beta carotene tablet equal to 25,000 IU, vitamin A."

"Sounds heavy."

"Maybe, but harmless."

"You can get all four in one tablet.

"You can and I may."

"All right," Will slaps the table. "Good stuff. Life span might not be inexorable after all."

"True, and fascinating," says Henry, "but I hope we can learn enough to get to the presently recognized life span."

"Oh no, Henry, think big!" Roddy laughs. "We really do need to wrap it up. See you next time."

"Hold on. I want to tell you about one new thing."

Henry draws out several sheets of a lined tablet paper. "I took these notes last week from a book I found at the university library. I was poking around while waiting to meet John Vana to go to the alumni council. My attention was caught by a word I'd never seen. From a Russian, V.V. Frolkis. He states, 'There are life-prolonging processes which take place along with the destructive processes of aging. Longevity and the life span depend on which one wins.' The fascinating word is *vitauct*. He invented it to describe the valiant warrior against the aging process. We do not know a whole lot about him--or her--but she's in there fighting for us all the time.

"Frolkis may be the first to suggest that there are 'life-prolongating mechanisms which come into place with age. There are various genetic theories, but he says these mechanisms come as aging advances. He called this vitauct, obviously from the Latin, 'vita,' life, and 'auctum'--to prolong.

"The mechanisms of vitauct, Frolkis suggests, are either genetically programmed, or somehow formed in relation to the self-regulation mechanisms of the body that are triggered by aging.

"Vitauct is the white hat--those things working for DNA reparation, perfection of gene regulation, gene redundancy, the protein-synthesizing system, the reproductive potential of the cells, augmentation of the antioxidant systems, among other things.

"Aging, on the other hand, is a band of bandits in the black hats--causing relentless DNA damage and alterations, detrimental shifts in the membrane-gene relationships, in genome regulation, in protein-synthesizing, among other things.

"I am over-simplifying. I saw that this book had been published in 1982 so I thought there must be a later Frolkis book. There was.

Just received. Published in 1991 with a co-author. It gets into evolution, and into related biological processes, and is just more complex and technical than suits our objectives.

"It is important to know their theory. I think it tells us that we should not quit trying to offset aging.

"Maybe this summarizes the concept: 'Vitauct is the biological process inherent in any living system; it stabilizes the organism's vital activity, prevents and liquidates many factors of aging, and increases life span.'

"For example--and I will not dwell on this--'The authors believe that aging is not genetically programmed'--but that genetic forces trigger other processes.

"They put aging on one side and on the other, they put vitauct. It is the ratio between aging and vitauct that determines the life span.

"So," says Roddy. "Like the mighty Mississippi flooding against the levees, eroding, endangering, eager to wash through, and to the battlements come the National Guard with sandbags, bulldozers, cutting channels, fighting the inevitable, holding off for another day and another flood. Ultimately the river will win, but the vitauct guardsmen have held it back as long as possible."

"Sure, and like a football game," says Joe. "The Vitaucts, last quarter, defending the goal, breaking up plays, forcing punts, stopping end runs, holding the line--and finally the Agings win because all the time the playing field slopes in favor of them. The Vitaucts can't win, but they can make the Agings fight for every inch."

"Very good, Joe."

"Doesn't it tell us in another way, Henry," asks Will Mack, "that the body is its own best doctor. It tells us that there are possibilities that scientists can find out more about vitauct, perhaps reinforce the elements that make it work, perhaps find ways to slow for much longer periods the unrelenting flow of old man river."

"Right. I thought it was a fascinating proposition. Vitauct. Life fights for life. It is great to know."

V.V. Frolkis quotes a colleague as saying human development--aging--is not a constant unwinding of the biological clock. There is also some winding."

"Did he tell us how to wind the clock?"

"No. The body self-regulates. He didn't offer a clock key. I suspect our surest course is general good health--our Big Four--including antioxidant supplements.

"Gosh, it's late," says Roddy, "It's time to break this up, Henry."

"I've got to go, too, but let me tell you one more thought. Frolkis quoted another scientist that gerontology should not be considered the study of aging, because that is negative, concedes defeat. Gerontology is, he contends, a science of life from the standpoint of its finite quality."

"Sure thing. You bet we are talking about how to live."

"And the quality of life."

"See you next Friday.

"Hold on. I want to read one more passage from the Johnson free radicals book, an article by Larry and Terry Oberley"

"'Another way to attack aging is to leave the longevity genes alone but to alter the cause of aging. If damage to mitochondrial DNA is the cause of aging, it should be possible to add back intact mitochondrial DNA. This could be done, for instance, by packaging the important components of the mitochondrial genome in an inactive virus vector. If new mitochondrial DNA could be added periodically, then only damage to nuclear DNA would control aging. This means the human life span could be expanded five to ten times. We believe this will be possible in the near future. It is time now to start planning for the social ramifications of aging extension. The effects on size of population would of course be immense. We urge that planning on this problem start with haste.'"

"Near future? Does he have his tongue in his cheek?" asks Rodney.

Sounds like it to me," says Will Mack. "Start planning with haste?"

"I think he is serious--maybe over-dramatic," says Henry.

"Living 500 to a thousand years," says Joe Zaroom. "Unbelievable!"

"I'd have to agree, Joe. See you next Friday..But who knows?"

Chapter Eight

HEAD TO TOE

*V*iolet brings Henry a cup of coffee. Only he and Lear have arrived.

"Mr. Henry," she says, "All this talk about men growing older. What about women? You leaving them out?"

"Now, Violet," Henry stutters, "Don't you worry about my leaving out women. I'm for equal rights. Our personal checks are printed 'Lottie G. and Henry Murphy,' and I support all of her causes for women."

"Bam, you don't need to give me a campaign speech. I'll vote for you. I just wondered if what you are saying applies to women."

"I hadn't thought about any differences. We got into all this because we six old buddies just got to talking about it, but we aren't leaving women out.

"I get so involved in the subject and I go over it all with Lottie, go over my notes with her the night before I report here to the fellows, and she laughs about the old goats trying to live forever. But she listens. She's interested. And we do things together now, like walking and leaving off French fried potatoes."

"I'm glad to hear that. I've cut out French fries."

"Health is health. What's good for men is good for women. The books I'm reading don't make many distinctions. There is one thing I've noticed, and it should be rectified. Not enough studies involve women. This applies to cardiac research, aging, and other areas. The universities and researchers need to correct this imbalance."

"Women live longer than men," says Lear. "We ought to be trying to find their secret."

"That's right, but women will benefit the same as men from a change in life style. Husbands and wives need to go about this together. Our Final Four fits women perfectly. They'll both benefit. The diet is important for both. Exercise is especially needed by women, because they are more susceptible to osteoporosis, and exercise strengthens bones as we have already learned, and women are more likely to lose calcium after middle age and need to watch for adequate calcium in their diets, maybe need calcium supplements. I like the idea of husbands and wives getting into healthy lives together. 'Grow old along with me! The best is yet to be. The last of life, for which the first was made.'"

"You hit a nerve there," says Violet. "I just want someone to start young along with me."

"We're all hanging in there to dance at your wedding," says Lear. "Everything we are talking about, Violet, as old man Ridenhour used to say, is 'ambidextrous.' Fits both ways, men and women."

Henry pulls a sheet from his pile of papers. "I do have a quote-- here it is--I was planning to use it when it fit. Dr. Erdman Palmore of Duke University, in a newspaper in February of 1991, pointed out the fact that women live longer than men, as Lear said. 'Part of this is caused by some sex-linked hormones that give women natural protection against some diseases, such as heart disease and stroke.'

"'But,' he writes, 'men could live longer by acting more like women!' How about that, Violet? This is true because 'about half the difference in mortality rates is caused by the more dangerous lifestyle of most men. Men die more often than women from accidents (reckless driving and dangerous occupations), homicide and combat (men are more violent), suicide (men use more violent means), lung cancer and respiratory diseases (men smoke more), cirrhosis of the liver (men are more likely to become alcoholic), and heart disease (men smoke more, have more cholesterol, have more hostility, etc.).'

"He concludes this observation by noting that men could increase their longevity by changing their lifestyles--eat wiser, fight less, imbibe less, stop smoking, drive slower, be calmer and less hostile--or, as Dr. Palmore put it, 'like women!'"

"That will never happen!" Violet snorts. "The one I'm working on has got most of those faults." She pauses. "But I figure I can straighten him out."

"Ah, the Violet treatment. Maybe that is the secret we've been looking for."

By now the others have arrived. Violet takes their orders.

They finish eating and push back their plates.

Henry chuckles and says, "How would you like to hear about a treatment where you laugh yourself to good health?"

"That will be a change from crying about diets and exercise," Will Mack answers.

"Norman Cousins, the distinguished editor of *The Saturday Review*, spent the last years of his life fascinated with the relation of mental attitude to illness and good health. As we study good health and long life, I think it's helpful, fun, for us to know about Norman Cousins.

"Cousins had a bout with death, won, wrote a short book telling how he helped his victory by laughing and joking. Incidentally, I got to know him when I was teaching."

"Cousins had come down with a rare disease that in time was ultimately diagnosed as ankylosing spondylitis. That's a disintegration of the connective collagen in the spine. The specialist gave him one in five hundred chances, but said he had never seen anyone recover. That shook up Cousins, as you might imagine, and he later wrote, 'Up until that time, I had been more or less disposed to let the doctors worry about my condition. But now I felt a compulsion to get into the act.'

"Good thinking," says Lear.

"Sure was. This disease is in the family of arthritis. Cousins had people at his magazine do some research for him and concluded that this illness had been activated when his collagen supply had been damaged by several exposures to undue amounts of carbon monoxide while in Russia on a trip from which he had just returned. His quick research convinced him that healthy body collagen depended on adrenaline and that to combat it his endocrine system, particularly his adrenal glands, needed to function fully.

"He further concluded that pain-killing drugs had a deleterious effect on the adrenal glands. So he concluded that even aspirin could be harmful in the treatment of collagen illnesses that he had."

"Aspirin harmful?" asks Victor. "They prescribe aspirin for arthritis."

"I know. Cousins takes issue with a lot of medical practices."

"He ought to," says Lear.

"Well, Cousins decided that he could stand the pain, but what would be done to reduce the inflammation that accompanies collagen disease? His research told him that vitamin C might activate the adrenal glands, which might reduce the inflammation. Shortly he was to take massive doses, and this vitamin, or something, had immediate effect on the flow of adrenaline.

"His doctor did not disagree, and apparently saw this self-diagnosis as a determined will to live, which he applauded. He might not have agreed with the medical validity, might have thought beneficial indications were a result of a placebo effect, but he knew the positive attitude of the patient was something a doctor desired. Besides there wasn't much hope otherwise.

"Cousins had previously concluded that emotional tension, frustration, and suppressed rage had a negative effect on the body chemistry."

"I've always thought that," said Will Mack, "always thought these things aggravated arthritis."

"I remember your saying so," Henry acknowledges.

"Cousins and his doctor concocted a program calling for the full exercise of the *affirmative emotions* as a factor in enhancing body chemistry. Then he hit on laughter, speculating that 'it was easy enough to hope and love and have faith,' but something more was needed to get the juices flowing.

"He obtained old movies of the Marx Brothers, films of Candid Camera, and others, and 'made the joyous discovery that ten minutes of genuine belly laughter had an anesthetic effect and would give me at least two hours of pain-free sleep.' The nurse read to him from humor books. He began to get better.

"Cousins put great store in the fact that his doctor, an old friend, 'encouraged me to believe I was a respected partner with him in the total undertaking. He fully engaged my subjective energies.'

"No question," says Victor, "that a doctor's respect for the patient's views--even dumb views--helps a lot. I know."

"Cousins was now fast approaching his final thesis: 'The chemistry of the will to live is a potent curative'; and 'I have learned never to underestimate the capacity of the human mind and body to regenerate. . . .'"

"That is his profound message, isn't it," says Will Mack. "Not laughter itself, but the attitude it brought."

"True. He is saying in so many words that the body has within it the power to cure itself, in many cases, and to assist in the cure in virtually all cases. He quotes Dr. Albert Schweitzer: 'Each patient carries his own doctor inside him. They come to us not knowing that truth. We are at our best when we give the doctor who resides within each patient a chance to go to work.'"

"I like Schweitzer," says Lear.

"So did Cousins."

"Laughter and vitamin C. I bet you don't learn that in a med school," says Lear.

"Remember," says Henry, "Cousins did not claim that laughter cures; although obviously he contends that vitamin C was the medicine, and laughter and good cheer were the magic that made the difference. Let me go on. Cousins quotes a notable medical researcher who says that ascorbic acid is not strictly a vitamin, but rather a 'liver metabolite.' I am ready to believe with Cousins that ascorbic acid plays 'a vital role in the healing process.' I also believe with Cousins that ascorbic acid plays a preventive role: As he says, 'The significance of ascorbate in the treatment of collagen diseases such as arthritis, therefore seems compelling.'

"It seems to me, Victor, that if it vitamin C is good treatment, it certainly follows that it is a preventive. I have begun to take a modest amount of vitamin C as a safeguard against arthritis, and in the tone of Cousins, a confident hope that I am not going to have gnarled fingers and arthritic pain in all my joints. But I am not going to get in the business of prescribing medicine for you birds."

"You may be on to something good," says Victor.

"Well, there is no known preventive for arthritis," says Roddy.

"I'm not prescribing, just reporting." Henry reiterates. "Vitamin C also serves as one of the antioxidants."

"Henry continues. "When Norman Cousins first wrote in a medical journal about his experience, he heard from three thousand doctors from around the world. He sums up their comments: ' . . . one of the main functions of the doctor is to engage to the fullest the patient's own ability to mobilize the forces of mind and body in turning back disease.' This is his main message. Norman Cousins wrote the book--it is *Anatomy of Illness*-- to let others know that the mind and body can take over healing in a manner that cannot be reached by drugs, medicines, and medical equipment."

"You had us spellbound, professor," Rodney says. "Wonder what the medical fraternity thinks about all that?"

"Many of them agree, maybe most of them, with the regenerative powers of mind and body. But read the book. This is a book that I definitely recommend. While I was at the library I scanned two other books by Cousins on this general subject. One is titled *The Healing Heart*, which tells about a later heart attack he suffered and how he coped with the fear and the doubts. The other is *Head First* and in it he arrays the scientific evidence to support the ideas and answer the questions raised in the book that I have just summarized. All three of these books are well worth reading."

"Now, Henry," Will Mack asks, "Is this message that the body can frequently heal itself if we will just let it?"

"That is the underlying premise, no doubt about it. And cheer it on, Cousins would add."

"Well, that is interesting," says Victor. I have long since come to the conclusion, out of my own experiences, none as dramatic as Cousins had, that most aches and pains would go away if you went about your business and ignored them. When a doctor has simply given me instructions to take an aspirin and call if the whatever-it-was didn't get better, I usually did not take the aspirin and I got cured anyhow."

"You got it right buddy," Joe Zaroom declares. "My daddy was from the old country. He said pain was something to be ignored, something to be greeted by contempt, something you should refuse to put up with. You could stare it down, he claimed."

"Now Joe, don't get carried away, don't forget that our Final Four includes counting on the doctor's regular advice,": says Will Mack.

"Oh he respected doctors. He just didn't respect pain."

"Let me put in a concluding word," Henry takes over. "I want to leave a couple of thoughts about Norman Cousins. I knew him and read after him for years when he edited the *Saturday Review* and I have been following his views on healing since they first hit the newspapers. He did not say that laughter cured illness. It took him several years to refute that charge. He said that pleasant emotions, old friends, an understanding family, love, and including fun and laughter, helped your body functions do their own good things, which a good doctor would also be trying to help your body to do.

"Neither did he suggest that the burden was on the patient to cure himself, but he did contend that the patient could play a big role, and he did embrace a maxim quoted in the introduction of his book on the heart: A 17th-century physician, Thomas Sydenham, declared, 'The arrival of a good clown exercises more beneficial influence upon the health of the town than twenty asses laden with drugs.'"

"Right on!" says Lear.

"But I have a sequel," Henry holds up his extended fingers. "Just by chance last night after I had all of my notes ready for today I picked up an old issue of *The Saturday Evening Post* because I saw an article entitled, 'The Laughter Prescription,' and to my surprise it had been written by none other than Norman Cousins. In the article he noted that the newspaper stories had made it appear that laughter was all there was to it, so he had then written the piece for the medical journal on which I've already reported.

"He said that he had made the point that his physician and he 'regarded laughter as a metaphor for the full range of the positive emotions.' That is what I told you he had said.

"But then he wrote: 'Perhaps I might have been a lot less defensive if I had known what I know now. Medical researchers at a dozen or more medical centers have been probing the effects of laughter on the human body and have detailed a wide array of beneficial changes--all the way from enhanced respiration to increases in the number of disease-fighting immune cells. Extensive experiments, working with a significant number of human beings, have shown that laughter contributes to good health. Scientific evidence is accumulating to support the biblical axiom, 'A merry heart doeth good like a medicine.'"

"Hospitals ought to post that in every hospital room," says Victor. "My nurse daughter says the worst thing about her job is cranky, complaining men."

"Good humor," says Will Mack. "I've always believed in it."

"In the article he cites several scientific experiments and a number of anecdotes to reinforce his premise, so he does put much more store in the power of hearty laughter than we might have been led to believe. He also told several jokes in this article but I'm afraid you have already heard them."

"Try us," says Will Mack.

"Well, this one may have missed you since he claims it is original. Cousins made a rather stilted speech before a prestigious audience, including his friend Bennett Cerf, a publisher and collector of jokes. Cerf advised him that he should lighten up and tell a funny story at the beginning of his speeches. 'Hasn't anything funny happened to you recently?'

"Yes, Cousins told him, 'I had spoken in Albany only a week earlier at a special meeting of the Board of Regents to welcome General Eisenhower in his new role as president of Columbia University. I sat next to General Eisenhower and tried to compose myself. . . . He leaned toward me and spoke in a whisper: "What's the matter? You look pale."'

"'I whispered back . . . so many educators in their university gowns is a little intimidating.'

"'Do as I do,' said General Eisenhower. 'Whenever I feel nervous before I speak I use a little trick . . . I just transfer my nervousness to the audience. . . I look out at all the people in the audience and just imagine that everyone out there is sitting in his tattered old underwear.'

"Bennett Cerf was entranced. 'Great, great! . . . The next time you speak, just begin your talk with the Albany story and the advice given you by General Eisenhower. . . . Two weeks later I spoke to a club in St. Louis and I began my talk with the Eisenhower anecdote. It didn't produce even a ripple. The audience was stony faced. The rest of my speech was uphill all the way.'

"Following the lecture a man came up to me. "The story about General Eisenhower. . . . Are you sure it happened to you?" I said, 'Of course it did.'

"'That's strange, he replied. 'Bennett Cerf lectured here last week and said it happened to him.'"

The fellows at the table chuckle.

"Well, good. I got more laughs than Cousins did. But not much."

"We didn't want to scare Violet. That's a pretty good story," says Will Mack.

"And that's a very good book report, Mr. Professor," Roddy slaps the table.

"Good cheer could help in more ways than healing," adds Victor. "All those mean-talking people in Congress and the TV talk shows ought to have to watch old Marx Brothers movies first thing every morning."

"Not bad public policy."

"See you next week."

Chapter Nine

Old Age Disease

*V*iolet takes their orders. "The cook says you gents are going to put hogs out of business. Nobody gets anything fried anymore."

"I weaken and sneak my fat later in the day," says Rodney.

" I have now checked out forty books and am just getting started. This has got me hooked. I'm glad we don't meet for breakfast every morning or I couldn't keep up. And they tell me at the office that I am neglecting my work."

"Work, Henry! What work?"

"You know I've got to keep them fooled--and on their toes--and cheered up. Young people tend to get discouraged when construction slows down--get scared. But I've seen building booms come and go. Cheer is one thing I can contribute so I don't have to back up for my paycheck."

"Henry, that reminds me," Roddy says, "I've been thinking about something that I believe has a lot to do with keeping fit as we grow old. I am not sure of the word--but I think it is 'spirit'--means a lot of things. Take things as they come, and move on. We've seen worse--whatever it is. Don't complain and don't give in. Keep looking for new things like you're doing with your book reports to us. Spirit."

"You're right, Rodney," says Will Mack. "The psychologists know it. Look to the future, be excited about what younger people around you are doing, about what is going on at City Hall, about what you are doing tomorrow, next week, this afternoon. Don't quit."

"I've got a little snippet on this card," says Henry, "from one of my favorites, *Aging Well* by James Fries: 'But to stay young you need, in certain senses, to act young. . . . enthusiasm is perfectly permissible. . . You are not old as long as you look forward with real anticipation to the future.'

"Entirely true. 'Play ball!' as the umpire yells. A sad day when you wake up with nothing to look forward to," says Joe. "Act young. Play ball!"

"Exactly," says Will Mack. "I told Ethel that when I die I want to be planning what I am going to do on the morrow."

"On the morrow! Now let me get back to my notes so we can put off that morrow as long as possible."

"Henry, have you covered all the chronic diseases?"

"No. I've got a lot of notes but it has been tempting to talk about other things.

"But I promised to talk about head to toe, Alzheimer's to gout. I'll do my best. But remember, I didn't ever intend to talk about disease and medical treatment. My assignment was to find out how to meet aging head on and with style."

"All right, Henry," says Victor, "what about Alzheimer's disease? I live with an overhanging fear that I'll go that way."

"I wish I could tell you what causes it. I wish I could tell you that there is a cure, even some treatment. I can only tell you that there is more research on Alzheimer's than ever before. Not enough. Best advice now, keep fit, keep active, keep caring about friends, keep interested in new ideas, projects, and activities--and pray."

"Henry," says Rodney, "it also requires advice and help to the spouse and family, so most medical centers dealing with Alzheimer's have special programs to help families cope."

"Yes, and families really need that help and advice."

"How do you know you have it? How do you know you are getting it?"

"I can tell you what to look for in Alzheimer's, but my assignment is to tell you what to do to avoid disease, and sadly, there is nothing I can tell you that will help you avoid Alzheimer's because they don't know what causes it.

"Let me paraphrase from an article in the *Handbook* edited by Birren and others, an article by Raskind and Peskind. The patient becomes disoriented and repetitious in conversation, eventually the patient may be unable to recognize family members, severe memory difficulties, and there are personality changes.

"It takes skillful medical diagnosis to determine that the disorders constitute Alzheimer's. According to Parhad and Rohs, the only definite diagnosis is by examining tissue from a brain biopsy or autopsy, although they can be ninety percent certain if some specified criteria are present."

"It's bad business. I hope they soon get a breakthrough in their research," says Rodney.

"I am sure they will. Just last month I read of a breakthrough at Duke's Alzheimer's Center." Henry flips several papers in his little notebook. Strittmatter and Allen Roses of the Joseph and Kathleen Bryan Alzheimer's Disease Research Center have discovered a likely culprit--a genetic risk factor that may predispose people to Alzheimer's."

"What does that mean?"

"Well, we can't be sure, but if it is genetic then the riddle is on the way to being solved.

"Gosh I hope so," says Victor.

"Dr. Roses predicts that maybe in time a pill can delay the onset of Alzheimer's disease."

"Come on! Can't be that simple."

"Good news."

"To move on," continues Henry, "mental illness, senility, and depression are likely to plague older people. These are serious matters and require medical attention.

"Well do we remember our good friend," says Roddy, "who was suffering from depression. We never guessed he would commit suicide. That is when I learned that depression is far more than simply being depressed. It can be an organic disease. Don't let your friends suffer deep depression without seeing a doctor. It is a chemical disorder that can be corrected."

"You're right. That is sometimes called clinical depression. But for some wise words of caution listen to Dr. Busse of Duke University. 'The depressive periods given attention in the longitudinal subjects were frequent, usually recurrent, and of short duration. Such depressive episodes can hardly be considered other than a feature of everyday living and should not be treated with antidepressants or other medication. Rather, supportive measures and the utilization of restorative activity which returns the individual self-esteem to an acceptable level is the best procedure to bring relief and reduction in frequency.'"

"Depression should not be ignored, you agree?"

"Agreed.

"Now I am not going to cover the catalogue of diseases and disabilities. I've picked a few that are likely to bother older people. I used two books--the American Medical Association *Family Medical Guide,* and Consumer Guide's *Family Medicine Guide.* There are a number of other such works.

"The eyes. Cataracts. One out of four people over 75 suffers cataracts. What to do about them? A regular eye exam. Caught in time, absent complications, the operation is routine. Another reason for regular exams is to identify glaucoma early. That could cause blindness. Early detection by regular exams and prompt medical attention. Now get this about vitamins. At a conference of the New York Academy of Science this year Allen Taylor reported in a paper that 'antioxidant nutrients, specifically vitamins C and E, and carotenoids . . . are probably preventive agents against light-induced cataract and age-related degeneration of the macula'--the center of the retina where your visual perception is most crucial."

"There you are, dammit!" Lear blurts. "Vitamins! Of course we need them!"

"We've already agreed we need anti-oxidant supplements?" says Will Mack.

"I agree. I'm not sure we all agree."

Roddy interrupts, "I can cover teeth." Charlie sent me a 1989 'Age Page.' Teeth can cause other diseases or disorders. Teeth need preventive care, frequent checkups, self-examination for bleeding or unusual conditions. We know to brush morning and night.

Flossing, use of fluoride in water or toothpaste or mouth rinses, removal of plaque by a dental hygienist. We should rinse with a mouthwash. A dental checkup can spot cancer and other problems. Preventive care. That's what we can do. Self-examination, one of our Final Four."

"Thanks, Roddy," says Will Mack, "and another important thing if you have a heart disorder, or heart murmur, or an artificial hip bone, or other internal irregularities, any dental work can cause dangerous heart or other internal infections. Like in that old song, the gums are connected with the hip bone and everything else. Make your dentist discuss all this before you sit down in his chair, even for a cleaning. Don't learn this the hard way."

"Very good," Henry claps his hands. "Let's get to diabetes, a killer if not controlled. It also contributes to cardiovascular, heart and lung diseases. To spot diabetes, have a regular exam. It is especially dangerous for older people. Get it treated before it gets out of hand. I can't tell you how to avoid it. It's hereditary in a third of the cases, and is related to pancreas dysfunctions. My mother used to threaten when I was about 10 years old that I would get diabetes if I didn't quit stealing from the sugar bowl, but nothing bad ever came of that. Obesity can be a cause of diabetes. Incidentally, I just read that obesity is the 'disease of all diseases.'"

"Ah, obesity, thy name is lack of will power," chants Rodney.

"Now, let's turn to the lungs," says Henry. "Emphysema. A terrible, relentless disease. Best way to avoid it is to stop smoking. That is not the only cause, but the big cause. Could sometimes be genetic. Could be air pollution. Talk to your doctor if short of breath, have lung congestion signs, too much coughing. You better avoid it, because there is no known cure.

"You can get a lung transplant," says Joe.

"Maybe, but that is a hell of a price to pay."

"Then," Henry picks up again, "there is cirrhosis. Gosh. Don't drink too much alcohol. Could also be caused by hepatitis, and some internal disorders.

"Now let me move down to diverticulitis and stomach or peptic ulcers. A lot of things cause an excess of stomach acids which cause ulcers. It is thought that too much alcohol, smoking, and medicine like aspirin, are some of the causes."

"I didn't realize it, Henry," says Victor, "but you can die from diverticulitis. A friend of mine, a Chicago Postal Inspector, is in intensive care. Ruptured diverticulitis. Did you know that could happen?"

"You're right. How do you avoid it? By consciously eating more bulk--cereals, fruits, vegetables. And drinking lots of fluid. Little pouches form outside the colon wall, called diverticula, caused by weakness in the wall or undue pressure from within. When they get infected or inflamed it is diverticulitis. Sometimes it is uncomfortable, sometimes painful, sometimes dangerous. If your annual physical includes an endoscopic examination, looking for polyps, they'll find the diverticula, which about one-third of people over 60 have. Better get the exam, and the doctor will prescribe.

"Finally, let me turn to gout, as I promised. This is caused by too much uric acid which crystallizes around joints, most likely the big toe, but could be at any joint. Rich living, they used to say. King Henry the Eighth's disease. Certainly an excess of alcohol could be a cause of the problem. Not likely to kill you. Ask your doctor what to do and what to quit doing.

"That is as far as I'm going. This is not a clinic or a medical school or a sick call. You ought to have a home medical book. I've mentioned two that I have."

"Thanks Henry," says Roddy. "I got through that list without developing too much hypochondria."

"There are a lot of other things that kill people or send them to the sick bed or make them invalids," says Will Mack. "I am thinking of some things that are not considered diseases, that I believe cause a lot of deaths. I don't need any doctor to confirm it. There is disappointment. There is boredom. There is loneliness. There is being broke. There is giving up."

"Right you are. A matter of spirit," says Victor.

"Life to many people is a passage through time, and little more," says Roddy. "They finish school and get a job and begin right then to look forward to when the children grow up and leave, when daddy can retire, and it seems to me even look forward to retirement, so even to the grave, as a successful goal. If the children leave and he doesn't lose his job and he gets his first retirement check and Social Security, he has won the race. He got there. But maybe the joy of each succeeding day passed him by, for he never did enter that game."

"I know quite a few like that. I don't know whether I can find any scientific evidence, but it seems to me that some people just waited to die, got ready to die, and then died. They ran out of purpose. Others seemed to look at each new day as the beginning of life, exciting, a time for learning and doing."

"No question about it," says Zaroom. "I've known people even in their fifties who seemed to feel they had done about all they were going to do. And generally they were right."

"Yes, what is the spark?" asks Victor. "What makes the difference? I wish I knew. The secret of staying young is staying young. Organ reserve may run out as Henry tells us, but we don't need to try to beat it to the finish line. The spirit of youthful outlook doesn't need to run out--ever."

"Don't quit!" Zaroom almost shouts. "I play Sousa's marches on the gramophone every morning while I exercise. Don't ever quit!"

"This is silly," Victor continues, "but I say to myself when I stumble or forget, 'Well, old boy, after all you are fifty years old.' That tends to explain or excuse my misstep. It justifies my little lapses. After all, a fellow fifty is entitled to some leeway. Now you know I am 71, but my little deceit reminds me that you are only as old as you feel, or admit. Admit is the better word. Many a morning I feel my years, all of them, plus some extra ones, for all the time I was run hard and put up wet, but when I verbally excuse the old man of fifty, it lifts a burden I can feel rise from my shoulders. I'm fifty years old; I've got fifty to go."

"That's great," says Will Mack, "I put a different spin on that. I walk, like Joe taught me, and I do dumbbells, sit-ups, and a few other things, every morning--well most every morning. As I lean up and stretch toward my toes, I say, 'Well here is the 18-year-old Olympic diver, folding into a jackknife dive, perfect form, graceful, agile, strong, coordinated, a perfect dive.' I'd probably fall off a diving board, if I dared walk out on one now. But the image braces me, I get up off the floor with a lilt and a lightness. I can see that athletic figure of a young diver, bending, graceful. It makes me feel young. Makes me ignore the pains. Just the pains of a young athlete in training."

"I take it you don't exercise in front of a mirror," Roddy chortles.

"Sounds great, but the Olympic games must come to an end," says Lear. "I've got to go to the 'Y.' Got a building campaign going and I'll be hitting up all of you."

"See you next week. Roddy is trying to find a special book. Ambition to live long is nothing new."

"What is it, Roddy?" asks Joe.

"Don't know. Haven't found it."

Chapter Ten

LONGEVITY NOT A NEW GOAL

Only Will Mack and Victor Beane have arrived, and Violet is pouring coffee. "Why, Mr. Mack, do all of you laugh about getting old? My mama says getting old sure beats the other choice. I hate to think about it."

"Don't think about it," says Victor. "You've got your living to do. Go do it--so when you get my age you won't have any regrets."

"I already have regrets."

"It's hard, Violet, for people to come to the end of the road," says Will Mack. "There is no time to go back and do it over. Everyone can think of lost opportunities. If I had just done this--taken that job--bought that land--too late now.

"Too late now. Sounds sad, but needn't be. Can be the happiest time of your life.

"I used to go down the Northeast River, first when I was a boy, by raft. I did this for years, then later with my boy and occasionally one of his friends. It was a wonderful, lazy trip, mostly floated, and talked, fished and didn't catch anything, camped on the sound when we got there. Took three days. The river runs through deep woods, mostly swamps. There are only four places where you can make a decent camp. When we would get to one we'd have to decide whether to take it or go to the next. Might be dark when we got to the next one. So we'd have to have a pow-wow to decide whether to camp.

"The boys would say, 'Guess right. We can't come back.' Once we passed up a campsite, it was lost to us forever. We had left that opportunity behind. The river flows on. We can't come back.

"Odd how a little thing like that can be a big lesson in life. I don't worry about what I might have done. It is behind me like that campsite. Go on to the next, and when they are all behind us, they are gone forever.

"But, Violet, there is the sound. We would stay there as long as possible. Wonderful campsite. Driftwood for a fire at night. Could fish and catch some. Could go swimming and exploring. Could just about do what we wanted to do. No pressure.

"The river flows on and we can't turn back upstream. Our life runs on. It is where we are that we can handle, not where we might have been."

"Well, Mr. Mack, "I'm looking for the first campsite. Hope I find a Brave, not a rattlesnake."

"You'll do all right, Violet, and Vic and I will make our last campsite the best of our lives, until the fire burns down and the sun rises, as it surely will."

"Here come Henry and Lear. We have a quorum," says Victor.

Joe Zaroom joins them and is poured a cup of coffee. All are there except Rodney Thomas, who rushes in clutching a tattered book and a handful of crinkled notebook paper, bouncing with enthusiasm.

"Henry, I found the book. It is sommm-thing! This copy was printed in 1903, but originally published about 1550!"

"Great, Roddy!" Henry turns to the group. "Roddy read about an ancient Venetian who lived to be over a hundred years old, and who wrote a book about how to grow old. Roddy thought it would be great to see what they were saying about aging more than 400 years ago. Tell us, Roddy."

"I called the university library yesterday and discovered there was such a book, so I drove up there and got it. Of course they did not have the original and I couldn't have read it if they had. The name is *The Temperate Life*, or translated *La Vita Sobria*, in Italian, Joe."

"I'm not Italian--I'm Lebanese!" snaps Joe.

"Whatever," Rodney laughs and pats Joe on the top of his baseball cap.

"The librarian said it could also be translated, 'The Sober Life.'"

"Good, good," says Lear. "Let's take the first title. I'd rather be temperate than sober."

"He wrote four discourses, the first when he was eighty-three and the last when he was ninety-five. I've made some notes and I've put some markers in the book.

"His name was Louis Cornaro, from Venice, and in time he was referred to as the 'Celebrated Venetian Centenarian.' He was of an illustrious family, and somewhat sickly.

"Here, let me read: 'I never knew the world was beautiful until I reached old age.' He was extremely wealthy, and his palace in Padua is still in existence. I am quoting now from the first discourse, telling why he wrote: 'I have seen many of my dearest friends and associates, men endowed with splendid gifts of intellect and noble qualities of heart, fall, in the prime of life, victims of this dread tyrant . . .'--intemperance he was talking about. 'Therefore,' he continues, 'to prevent so great an evil for the future, I have decided to point out, in this brief treatise, what a fatal abuse is the vice of intemperance, and how easily it may be removed and replaced by the temperate habits of life. . . .'"

"Even then," snips Lear, "they were claiming that it's easy to change habits."

"Old Louis goes on to say he had been pressed to write by a number of young men who had seen their fathers die in the flower of life, 'while they behold me still hale and hardy and flourishing at my great age of eighty-three years.' I suppose life expectancy then was about twenty-five, or less. So these young people had urged Cornaro to tell them how he had been able to reach old age."

"Just like Henry telling us youngsters how to grow old," Zaroom quips.

"Not quite," answers Henry. "I'm the youngster reading to old coots."

"Well, to move ahead," Rodney says, flipping pages, "old Cornaro wrote, 'Now, Nature does not deny us the power of living many years.' He went on, 'dire infirmities from which I constantly suffered' caused 'my renouncing the errors of intemperance to which I had been very much addicted.'

"He was in terrible shape, not then forty years old. Here is what he wrote: 'The excesses of my past life, together with my bad constitution--my stomach being very cold and moist--had caused me to fall prey to various ailments, such as pains in the stomach, frequent pains in the side, symptoms of gout, and, still worse, a low fever that was almost continuous. . . . This evil . . . condition left me nothing to hope for myself, except that death should terminate my troubles and weariness of my life. . . .'"

"Terrible shape, terrible, and gout, too. I've had a little gout but I didn't want to die," Victor interrupts. "How did the old boy recover?"

"Ah, yes. The doctor's advice. Old Luigi--that's Italian for Louis, Joe, although his friends probably called him Alvice, the old Venetian name--was about gone from this world. He wrote, 'My physicians declared there was but one remedy left for my ills--a remedy which would surely conquer them, provided I would make up my mind to apply it and persevere patiently in its use!'"

"There you go," says Lear, "same old stuff--persevere--will power--I thought you had the ancient, magic potion. Easy to take. No sweat."

"That's right. The bad news is that the 'remedy was the temperate and orderly life, which . . . possessed as great strength and efficacy for . . . good results, as . . . an intemperate and disorderly life . . . for doing harm.'

"'In a word,' he wrote, 'I grew most healthy, and have remained so from that time to this day.'

"Now what did he do? Let me read from several places. '. . . I chose only such wines,' he said, 'as agreed with my stomach, taking of them only such quantity as I knew it could easily digest. . . .'"

"Good start,!" says Lear. "Henry, can't we add wine to the Final Four?"

"Proceed, Mr. Thomas."

"Okay. Cornaro went on, 'I observed the same rule with regard to my food, exercising care both as to the quantity and the quality. In this manner, I accustomed myself to the habit of never fully satisfying my appetite, either with eating or drinking--always leaving the table well able to take more.'"

"That's what they say," Joe Zaroom chimes in. "The best exercise is pushing away from the table."

"True, true, and as ancient Cornaro put it, 'I acted according to the proverb: "Not to satiate one's self with food is the science of health.""'"

"Well, damn," moans Victor, "Don't eat, don't eat."

"He had some other rules," Roddy continues. "I've picked them out to read them one by one:

"Guard against 'great heat and cold. . . .'

"Guard against 'extreme fatigue. . . .'"

"I'm for that," says Will Mack. "Never stand if you can sit down; never sit if you can lie down."

"Guard against 'excesses of any nature. . . .'

"'I have never allowed my accustomed sleep and rest to be interfered with. . . .'

"'I have avoided remaining for any length of time in places poorly ventilated. . . .'

"I've been 'careful not to expose myself too much to the wind or the sun. . . .'

"'I have also preserved myself . . . from those other disorders from which it is more difficult to be exempt; I mean melancholy, hatred, and the other passions of the soul, which all appear greatly to affect the body.'"

"Norman Cousins would have liked that."

"Good advice," says Victor Beane. "I can take care of the passions of the soul easier than the passions of the stomach."

"Okay, Vic. This one's for you, a proverb that Cornaro approved: '*Whosoever wishes to eat much must eat little*,' meaning, he explains, the eating of little prolongs life for many years of eating.

"And here is another one for you, Vic--and me," Rodney pats his ample girth. "'*The food from which a man abstains, after he has eaten heartily, is of more benefit to him than that which he has eaten.*'"

"He didn't realize he was reducing his number of free radicals."

"Right, and when pressed for details of how much he ate, Cornaro reported that his family had urged him to eat more, 'so that, while, with bread, the yolk of an egg, a little meat, and some soup, I had formerly eaten as much as would weigh in all exactly twelve ounces, I now went so far as to raise the amount to fourteen ounces; and, while I had formerly drunk but fourteen ounces of wine, I now began to take sixteen ounces.' These new amounts upset his system so he went back to the lower measurements.

"Drank more than he ate? Not a bad plan," says Lear.

"He did furnish a little leeway on diet. In the later part of his discourse, he admitted, 'I eat veal, kid, and mutton; I eat fowls of all kinds, as well as partridges and birds like the thrush. I also partake of such salt-water fish as the goldney and the like; and, among the various fresh-water kinds, the pike and others.

"A partridge would be two or three meals for him," says Will Mack.

"At another point he wrote, 'No one need feel obliged to confine himself to the small quantity to which I limit myself; nor to abstain from fruit, fish, and other things which I do not take. For I eat but little; and my reason in doing so is that I find a little sufficient for my small and weak stomach. Moreover, as fruit, fish, and similar foods disagree with me, I do not use them. Persons, however, with whom these do agree may--nay, should--partake of them; for to such they are by no means forbidden. That which is forbidden to them and to everybody else, is to partake of food . . . in a quantity so large that it cannot be easily digested; and the same is true with regard to drink.'"

"He didn't say anything about cigarettes--there were some habits they hadn't learned. But what about exercise?" Henry Murphy asks.

"As a matter of fact he did not seem to care much about exercising. He wrote in several places that he was frail and had a small stomach. He placed all of his bets of limited food and drink."

"He might have lived to 110 if he had exercised," Joe says.

"I suppose he got enough vitamins from those little thrushes, but he seems to have shorted himself on vitamin C by not eating fruits."

"He didn't know about vitamins, but it was amusing to find that he was in tune with Norman Cousins on a couple of points. And, he did not trust doctors and medicine too much."

"I'm with him on that," says Lear.

"One time when he had suffered injuries, perhaps broken bones, and had developed a fever, the doctors were called in. Cornaro wrote, 'convinced that the regular life I had led for many years had united, equalized, and disposed all my humors so well that they could not possibly be subject to so great alteration,' he 're-fused either to be bled or to take any medicine. I merely had my arm and leg straightened, and permitted my body to be rubbed with certain oils. . . without using any other kind of remedy, . . . I entirely recovered--a thing, which . . . seemed to my doctors nothing less than miraculous.'"

"Good grief," says Will Mack, "the *cardinal humours*? We ought to study that, Henry. I bet they are coming back in style."

"I wouldn't doubt it but I hope bleeding with leeches doesn't come back," says Henry.

"Why don't you check for a book, Henry? Ben Jonson wrote a comedy about humours about the time Louis Cornaro was doing his writing."

"You fellows come back to earth. I was saying Cornaro appeared to agree with Cousins some four hundred and fifty years earlier. He seemed to sense, and then be convinced, that the body could generally take care of itself, that orderly living 'is the true and only medicine.' He continued this thought: 'Since, then, a man can have no better doctor than himself, and no better medicine than the temperate life, he should by all means embrace that life.'

"Well, friends, that is the story and advice of the celebrated Venetian Centenarian, who says, when we are all through that the best food is what you leave on the table.

"I conclude with his words." Roddy raises his hand in mock benediction. "'O holy and truly happy Temperate Life, most worthy to be looked upon as such by all men! . . . O most holy and most innocent Sobriety, the sole refreshment of nature, the loving mother of human life, the true medicine both of soul and of the body; how much should men praise and thank thee for thy courteous gifts!'"

"Amen and amen," intoned Will Mack.

"Roddy, extremely in-ter-resting," says Joe. "This ain't a new subject."

"Good going."

"Oh holy temperate life." Lear shakes his head.

"Thanks, Roddy."

Victor Beane raises his hand, as if to interrupt before Henry moves to leave. "One of the things we haven't talked about, as such, is death. We've been talking about extending health that's good. But don't older people have to come to terms with death?"

"I suppose so," says Lear. "I don't think about it except to dismiss it. It's a matter of fate. In the war, I knew death could come any minute. Leave it to fate."

"Me too, Lear," Will Mack says, "I dodged fate, too. Odds were I might get Jerry's bullet. But I didn't need to believe it. The other feller, not me. I was certain I'd get out alive. So did 'most everyone else, including those who got killed. Now, fifty years later. Another story. Not fate any more. It is a sure bet. The Reaper will get me."

Rodney had recovered from his book review. "That's not the point. That's not what scares us. Of course we are all going to die. I accept that. I'm ready for it. Our problem. . . ."

Zaroom interrupts. "Like Pope John said, 'My bags are packed.'"

Roddy continues. "Well, mine are packed too, I think, but I sure haven't zipped them up yet. Our problem, as I was saying, is not that we will die, but how will we die? If we could be sure of promptness and dignity, I think we'd have a lot less fear of death. I worry more about whether I will linger in comatose, or worse, be aware but totally incapacitated. I want to be clipping roses in my garden when I go--but I must say, preferably about thirty years from now."

"More and more people are thinking that." says Will Mack. "Sherwin Nuland has written a best seller, *How We Die*, observing, among many other thoughts, that people don't want hi-tech dying by extending living beyond the reasonable time for death. You can plan how you want to be let alone to die in peace."

"That's the thing," Vic Beane says. "I've got all the legal documents. Suppose they don't follow my wishes to be unhooked.. I've talked to my children and my wife and my doctor and my lawyer, and now I am talking to you, my friends. Don't let me linger. Don't interfere with the Lord's work."

Joe Zaroom has appeared anxious, uneasy with this conversation. "Okay, okay, sure. We'll jerk your plugs out. I've signed the papers, too. But what do you want us to do when you get batty and senile, don't know where you are most of the time? You lie there in bed with your mouth hanging open, snorting and snoring, raising hell about your soup being too cold or your egg too hard, wetting your bed, and running everybody crazy. How are you going to write out instructions to take care of that?"

Victor Beane squirms. "Joe, that's what scares me. I don't know how to handle it. I've always said that when I die I want to be painting the house or planting the garden."

"Right," says Will Mack. "I don't want an irritable invalid to be the last picture my grandchildren and children have of me. I don't want to put my wife through that ordeal."

"I remind myself," Victor continues, "that I may get old and feeble, but I'm not going to turn irritable and irascible."

"You're already irascible."

"Maybe the time comes when you don't have much control of your feelings and actions," Victor goes on. "Maybe the dread, the constant little pains, the frustration of your damnation, make you something you haven't been and don't want to be. Maybe you're cussing not your keepers, but your fate that consigned you to an invalid's bed instead of cutting you down in the rose garden."

"Now, hold on," says Henry. "Sure all of that is frightening, but that is what we are talking about: How to reach the end of our days in walking health. It can be done."

"I believe you. How to run out the string while running."

"You're on the money," says Rodney. "And we do have to break this up. I've got a client waiting."

Will Mack stands up. "I've come to the rationalization that I have a longer life expectancy now than I had when I was fifty. Statistics bear me out. Then I prepared for immediate death by getting enough insurance to protect my family. I had a will prepared. I more and more realize that I could have died or been killed, by accident or by design, in war or on the highways, by a heart attack or cancer, so daily we have faced death.

He sits down, as he continues to talk.

"With all of that, I was preparing for the chance death, but now it is something else. It is no longer chance I am facing. It is certainty. Even if I am lucky, death is out there waiting. I can accept that calmly. It is not beyond the horizon--we can look at it. What is my image of death? It could be a vicious black bear with great claws and jaws, but for me it is a loving shepherd ready to embrace me and warm me, a shivering child, within the folds of his cloak."

"Thank you, Will. That's beautiful."

Rodney pushes back in his chair. "Last night I was watching on TV a Katherine Hepburn flashback of her movies and career-- Spencer Tracy and their nine pictures together--*The African Queen* and Humphrey Bogart. Great careers. All over. And I am watching and I remember all of those pictures, the names if not the plots, or the plots if not the names. I was there. My career, my time here, trailed theirs by a few years. All a reminder that the years are passed. They are at the end and I am trailing closely, all too closely. What did they achieve? What have I achieved? What have we achieved? What is the purpose of being here?"

"You make a difference," says Will Mack. "I'm not talking about a Churchill difference. Not many do that, and I'm not talking about a Mafia difference.

"You ought to be able to say that you helped upgrade society a bit, that you refreshed the atmosphere, that some part of the world is a little better.

"There is a little machine you can buy from one of these technology mail order firms. You turn it on and it sucks in air and blows it out clean. It doesn't worry about the world. It doesn't worry about all outdoors. It refreshes the air, removes the impurities right there where it is. We can stand for fairness. We can be honest. We can recoil at injustice, perhaps some of us can be in a position to resist and rectify injustices. If we purify what we breath- -that is do the right and honorable thing where we are--we have then made a difference.

"You do the best you can," Rodney goes on. "Like Hepburn, you make the most of it. There is not much in looking back except for the joy of it. You play your role, and that's that. And so be it. It is so with everyone. Life starts, it stops. There is no continuity, no logic, no fairness guaranteed, much luck."

"I knew a man who struggled to accumulate a fortune because," says Will Mack, "he told me he wanted to establish a dynasty. I suppose a man could think establishing a dynasty is a way of doing the impossible, of existing beyond death. That seems to be important to some. He saw in his fortune, if he had made one, an extension of his life, a carrying on. But it is not so. I am proud of my son. He is going so well. He is a better man than I. He could be snatched away by any number of instruments of fate. It would all be over. My dynasty would be finished before it was started.

"There was Spencer Tracy marching across Africa. I am marching here, with millions of others. My son is back there somewhere. We are together in space but not in time. Einstein explained that, if you read him with an open mind."

"My son is here and he is not here. He is not me. He cannot pick up my body and carry it, he cannot enter it and become me, and that is not to be regretted. There is no dynasty. The present may acclaim the man for glory or position or advantage, but it doesn't matter, couldn't matter, to the ancestor.

"We march along, some briskly, some warily, some dancing, falling, sliding sideways, but relentlessly marching. Maybe it is the moving sidewalk, like in the airports, carrying us somewhere just because we stepped on it. More than marching across the desert set, it is as if the set were on a revolving belt moving under us, and we are simply keeping up and some stumble, some quit and sit down, and are carted back off the left of the stage. The goal is to march, head up, off the right of the stage. It is my life for a period of time, no longer.

"I take pride in my son, but I cannot expect him to fulfill my destiny, no matter what dynasty I built for him. He has to get there on his own. These are two lives. I remember my father in that distant day. These were three lives. Across a whole century. I remember my grandfather in an even more distant day. When we die, it is not dynasty that is important. It is, if anything, legacy. And that is simple. Don't ask if they built castles for their dynasty. Ask if they did their best, were fair and honest and kind. That's legacy.

"I have carried on my march. It has been up to me. I have got to finish it in style. . . ." Will Mack pushed back his chair, as if to leave.

There were tears in Rodney Thomas's eyes. "I never talk about this, as each of you know, my boy died when he was eight years old, smart, happy, beautiful. I was in a bottomless pit and there was no use to come out. His mother was down there with me, too.

"It wasn't the link to the future that mattered. It was the joy that had gone out of my life. I cursed God. He had damaged me, wounded me beyond recovery, taken away the sunshine and the reason for living.

"I couldn't do anything for his mother and she couldn't do anything for me. Poor thing, she had lost more than I had.

"If there had been your moving stage, Will, we would have laid there and let it cart us off. We laid there a long time and the Lord let us be until we were ready to get up.

"I quit my job. Lost it I suppose. And when I got up, I wanted somehow to make my little boy's life count for something. I wanted his childlike faith in me to be true. Every day since I got up from that devastation, I have tried to make my life worth his. I live on his legacy. I've turned my back on some good deals, I've turned aside from some easy money, I've gotten up in the middle of the night to help somebody. Some people's fathers, or mothers, make them a better man. There is a generational connection. My little boy made me a better man."

Chapter Eleven

MEMORY AIN'T SO BAD AFTER ALL

*V*iolet was there with her order pad, everyone had arrived, and all had been served coffee.

"We've got six kinds of dry cereal. I'll name them if you want me to. We've got a pot of oatmeal for Mr. Beane and anybody else who wants it. I've got orange, grapefruit, prune, apple, and tomato juice. I've got whole wheat bread. I've got no strawberries, but I've got bananas. I've got acidophilus milk. I've got yogurt. This is Healthville unlimited. So order up."

Lear is first. "Can I have butter--excuse me, oleo--on my oat-meal?"

"You can have whipped cream if you want it. What's going to happen to our short order cook if all of you turn into health nuts?"

"Don't knock it," says Rodney, "I've already lost 10 pounds."

"Yea, don't forget I get ten dollars if you haven't lost 20 pounds by Thanksgiving," says Violet.

"I know. Don't count on it for your Christmas money. I'll make it."

"Remember my deal, Violet," drawls Lear, "Every cigarette you jerk out of my mouth you get a dollar."

"Smoke 'em up, Mr. Jones, I'm ready."

She takes the other orders.

Henry begins, "Today we want to talk about mentality and aging, and I can tell you something right off the bat about mental capacity. Older people get a bum rap. Except for physical illness and disease, which might apply to any age, older people still have their marbles."

Will Mack agrees, "It's the myths again, Henry. The conventional wisdom is that old people can't remember, can't learn, can't pay attention."

"Well I can't, or didn't remember names as well as I used to," says Joe Zaroom. "Bothered me. Used to know every person who came in the store a second time. Never forgot a name or a face. I was over at the VFW hut for a thing several months ago, and later that night I suddenly realized I couldn't recall a single new name, and I must have met twenty, thirty new people. Am I getting senile, I thought? Still, I remember the names of my ball players, and their parents too.

"I found a book about memory. Bought it long ago. I opened it and my eye fell almost at once on the reason. There was the stuff about linking images, making pictures and rhymes to remember names. I know all that stuff. That was not my problem. I saw this sentence, 'You must care about people.'

"That was it! I'm not losing my memory. I just didn't care whether or not I knew all those young veterans of Korea and Vietnam. I didn't need to know them. I needed to know my customers. I need to know my ball players. I just didn't much care what were the names of the young vets. They all knew me. That was enough."

"You are exactly right, Joe," says Roddy. "I hadn't thought about it, but I already know enough people. It's time to rest my mind. Damn! That's bad!"

"Right," says Zaroom. "After I read that one sentence, 'care about people,' I was ashamed. I ought to care about people. They are interesting. I would pretend they would be my customers, or had come to see my ball club, or have something to tell me I need to know. And you know, it's working.

"Also, Henry, I've got another book and some stuff I can tell you about, when you want me to."

"You're on target, Joe. The experts support you, more or less. Let's come back to your other book. I have looked at a lot of articles, and I can read between the lines that even the scientists doing the experiments can't quite immediately overcome the myth. They have a bias that tells them they are going to find older people not alert, not thinking, not remembering.'

"Found a good book called *Aging and Human Performance*, edited by a chap from the University of Waterloo in Canada, by the name of Neil Charness. Remember that name, Joe. I'll ask you later."

Zaroom comes right back. "Neil Charness is in the harness. I see a Royal Canadian mountie, red jacket, in the harness, Charness in the harness, with the horse holding the reins, and the horse yelling, 'What's the deal, Neil?' I'll tell you the Canadian's name next year."

"Not bad, Joe Boy. This book has articles about attention, remembering, comprehension, and problem solving. I'll sum them up.

"I called the university library and they sent it. I told the young lady what it was about, and asked her if she thought she could remember to send it, and quick as a wink she said, 'I'm worried you won't remember where you got it.' Her name is Violet White, Joe."

"You mean they trust you with a book, and mail it to you?" Joe laughs. "White paper of a library book. Violet your color when you lose the book. Violet White."

Very seriously, Henry nods, "Remember I was a faculty member seven years. They know me. I keep in touch. I'd still be there, I often think, if my uncles hadn't died in the same year. Family. But there I go, talking about what might have been. A sign of old age."

Henry brightens. "But I love it here. I wouldn't know all of you, if I hadn't come home. I'm lucky. I've had a good life."

"Good life, so far," Roddy corrects. "We're working on thirty more years."

"And I might yet write the great American novel. But let's get back to our classroom.

"The first topic is about attention. The two psychologists, one from the University of Maryland and the other from Syracuse University, 'view attention as the capacity or energy to support cognitive processing.'"

"Cognitive processing!" Victor Beane interrupts: "Suppose I said attention was reading or watching or listening without letting your mind wander?"

"They might buy that. I will. But they would test to see if your non-wondering mind was processing the information."

Victor asks, "Well, might the professors note that you could have the capacity, but not the energy, or have the energy but not want to use it? Sometimes when you are listening to somebody talking you are lucky if your mind can wander back to when you were a kid fishing in North Fork."

"My mind always wanders when I'm listening to a speech, but let's look at the scientific approach and results. Now I read all this very carefully, and I studied it along with some other works and made notes and little charts. Mostly it is good news, but if I read you all of their professional terms you would quit paying attention to me, and think about fishing, and rightfully so."

"Try us."

"For example, and I read, 'In sum, attention can be conceptualized parsimoniously as a single, global capacity providing the energy to support cognitive functioning.'

"Huh? You tried us!"

"I thought you'd enjoy that. Then they offer a less obscure comment, 'information processing is limited by a unitary attentional capacity.'"

"Yes, clear as a bell."

"Let me translate in my mother tongue. The researchers are trying to measure your alertness to what is going on around you, and your quickness in reacting to what you see or hear.

"The question is, does this mental attentiveness, this mental process of knowing what's up, slow down with age? They have figured out various laboratory ways to measure the reaction time to grasp and recognize something.

"For example, they get old people and young people to call out the color of the ink when they flash a card. The word 'red' might be printed in blue and if you call out red, you missed that one. They measure accuracy and time.

"They want to know if older people can process what they see. Does this capacity of the human mind slow down with age?"

"And does it?" asks Rodney. "Tell us. My attention span is waning."

"Yes. Your capacity to process information slips. You are slower in reacting, in sorting out, in identifying, in concluding. You may be more accurate, or as accurate, or sometimes less accurate, but you are slower.

"I don't believe I'm slower," says Victor.

"How much slower?"

"Ah, there's the catch. They have to infer how your mental process is working on the basis of some overt action you take. They note that 'there is debate over whether or not speed-accuracy trade-offs change with advancing age.'

"But," says Rodney. "You might not get less accurate even if you get slower?"

"That is roughly the final conclusion."

Henry continues, "They talk about global capacity, that you can pay but so much attention to all things going on around you. They conclude that the capacity to select, process, respond to what you see, hear and feel gets slower with age.

"You are more easily diverted from your task by extraneous events that intrude. I could have told them that without all the complex experiments.

"Then, again, in the same book, one experimenter expresses doubt about some of these conclusions of slowness with advancing age in some of the situations.

"This book could be the text for a semester's course. It took me a week to find time to get through it.

"I learned a lot about effortful versus automatic information in processing, selective attention, and more other things than I need to recount to you. You can read the book if you need to know more than I am telling you.

"Let me quote Alex Comfort: 'There is no overall intellectual decline with age. In general, with good physical and mental health and adequate intellectual stimulation, it appears that intellectual abilities do not decline. In fact, judgment, accuracy, and general knowledge may increase.'"

"Boy! Read that again," says Joe.

"My final conclusion is generally good news. Sometimes the older person is just as quick, most of the time a little slower, but all of these reaction time differences are measured in milliseconds.

"For example, in one of the unfavorable comparisons, the younger read a letter in the display in 60 milliseconds, the older read it in 85 milliseconds, with 20 and 35 milliseconds, respectively, for each additional letter. Those measurements are about typical."

"So," says Lear, "the final word is, what the hell is 25 milliseconds between a grandfather and his grandchild? There is a difference, but it ain't much."

"That's right," says Victor, "both could decide to run for the train if they saw it pulling out of the station, and if grandpa missed it, it would be that he couldn't run as fast, not that he didn't think to start quick enough."

"Is it fair to conclude, Henry," asks Roddy, "that there may be a little bit slowing down in processing a thought, but not enough to make a federal case out of it?"

"I'll buy that," says Henry.

"Now, Joe, let's talk about memory--what the experts call 'episodic memory--that is, memory for personally experienced events on activities." I'm drawing on Donald H. Kausler in the Charness book for this information. In the laboratory testing of memory, memory can be divided into five components: First, remembering lists; second, meaningful discourse; third, performed activities; fourth, the setting, time, sequence, place, etc., of some event; and fifth, things to do.

"I am not capable of describing how memory works--and perhaps no one else is--but memory is a fascinating subject. The event, thought, or comments go sometimes intentionally and sometimes unintentionally from the initial imprint, blended with whatever is already known about the language and the world, to a working memory, at which place it can be rehearsed or related to something else, and from where it might be moved deeper into more permanent storage--or it might be dismissed or disregarded, and lost.

"It takes no effort to remember permanently someone drawing a knife on you and barely missing your gullet. You might have to press your memory to hold this episode if you merely read about it.

It might be retained automatically, at least for a short-term if you saw it on the screen.

"If you made an effort to remember a name and face, a quote, a grocery list, a recipe by relating it to some image, you move the item beyond the temporary impression. If you relate a future task, such as stopping for a dozen eggs, or telephoning Jim, or something obvious, you will have put that future chore into at least your short-term memory.

"Then getting the information out of memory when needed is the ultimate proof. The more ways it is indexed, the more likely you are to recall it.

Lear says, "Good going. Like moving items into our warehouse. Some make it to a bin, but we haven't put its location on the inventory list. So we can't find it. Some we just neglect to put on the conveyor belt, and they never make it, carried away with the trash.

"Sure," says Rodney, "the question is do we become less able to put stuff on the conveyor, less likely to tag it for a bin, or do we just find that old age makes it difficult to search the warehouse?"

"Well," says Henry, "those comments don't do too much violence to the concept. Let me tell you some conclusions. So far, it has been demonstrated that there are some memory differences between young and older adults. But what are the reasons for this? And what is the practical effect?

"These components or memory are difficult to test in a laboratory setting. Dr. Kausler, who analyzed many such experiments, has observed that many elderly people who worry about their loss of memory 'simply forget how imperfect episodic memory is even for young adults.'"

"Sure," says Victor. "The big thing we are likely to forget is how forgetful we were when we were younger."

Henry chuckles. "That's about right, Dr. Karsler concludes, 'the capacity of working memory is assumed to decrease from early to late adulthood,' and he points out that 'Direct recall requires considerable cognitive effort, and is therefore likely to be somewhat more proficient for young adults than for elderly adults. The diminished capacity of working memory for conducting an active search of the stored contents is the probable reason for the age difference.'

"My conclusion is that we just no longer bother to store everything, and don't try too hard to search. Our memories are not all that bad. We just don't fully use them. And, I believe, there are ways for us to improve what seems to be bad memory."

Says Joe, "Right. Sure we can. Like in a lot of other things, we get sloppy, don't bother, like we don't exercise."

Beane says, "Same thing. I can meet a person now, and unless I've engaged him to fix my plumbing or my car, I don't trouble myself with his name. I can do better than that."

"Sure you can. Now, Henry," says Joe, "I had two more reports. I've already mentioned one. I read a piece about memory by Kent Collins who writes the "Golden Age" syndicated column. He referred to a book by Alan S. Brown so I bought it.

"Then I got a series of tapes--not books, about memory by Robert Montgomery.

"Now I am forcing myself to practice remembering. It is now one of my hobbies. Put tags on the stuff you put in your memory bins--some connecting link to help you find it when you want it. Make funny pictures to prompt your thought, write it down so you can see it."

"Brown, who is a professor at SMU, says memory isn't necessarily worse in old people, that we just worry about it more."

Henry says, "Well, Joe, you've got something there, I do believe. I find my memory spotty. Is it because we have become blasé? Is it because we are not motivated to remember?"

"All of that sounds reasonable to me, Henry," says Will Mack. "I believe our memory is not as bad as we old folks say it is. I believe your reports tell us that.

"Second, as Joe says, we can do something about it."

"Let me read from one of my little cards," says Henry. "The Vickery and Fries book--which I suggest you own and keep as a reference--tell us that jogging the memory is like jogging the legs and body. Memory needs exercise. There is short-term memory and long-term memory. When we learn a new name, it is placed in our short-term memory and soon replaced by something else. It must be placed in our long-term memory before it is lost. This is when memory problems with aging are most pronounced. There is difficulty in storing new information in long-term memory."

"Well, how do you handle that?" asks Victor.

"The same way you go up dark stairs. Concentrate on what you are doing at each step. Repeat the thing to be remembered--associate it with something--recall it to see that you have it. Be more deliberate in examining the item, to use Lear's warehouse analogy, tag it deliberately, and deliberately put it on the conveyor belt. Then call it back up to be sure it got in the right bin. As they say, if we don't use it, we will lose it."

"Or," Joe adds, "Use your brain or see it drain."

"Ugh."

"So," laughs Henry, "that's the gospel. For practical, everyday purposes, weak memories don't need to be a big problem of getting older."

"I want to give a quick report on one more book, just summarizing what we have talked about. The book was edited by James Birren and others, and I am going to quote mostly from a chapter by Judith Sugar and Joan McDowd.

"As to memory and learning, what they say is good news. They point out the difficulty of relating laboratory experiments to real life.

"They report that aging does not bring about a uniform decline in memory, that the differences in cognitive abilities favor the younger but only slightly, and 'from a practical point of view, observed differences due to age may be insignificant, though theoretically interesting.' Next, the differences can disappear after training and practice, and finally, 'on some memory and learning tasks, older adults sometimes simply perform better than some younger adults.'"

"That's a reassuring book," says Will Mack. I'm sure glad you discovered it."

"They also report that older people are more self-conscious about memory lapses, and this has an effect on laboratory performance. Older people also compare their memory with their ability to remember when they were younger--and here is some proof of bad memory."

"Cheer up," says Roddy. "Your memory was never all that good!"

"Exactly!. They have a little section entitled 'Everyday Memory and Aging,' and tell us when it comes to remembering things to do, prospective memory, the older person does better on this everyday activity."

"They also make the point that memory can be improved by training, by writing it down, and by practice. They did report, Joe, that 'older adults did not like bizarre images to remember paired associates."

"That may be. But I do. You need some image to associate before you put it in the bin."

"The older citizen also does better in regard to everyday lapses of attention. So, mark it down. Older citizens can be about as sharp as they want to be by practice and concentrating on what he or she wants to remember."

"We just have to care enough to remember," says Joe.

"I've just remembered I'm meeting an old client," says Roddy. "He won't forget to be there. He's 82 years old."

"See you next Friday. We will have a symposium on exercise and physical fitness."

"Symposium?"

Chapter Twelve

EXERCISE--TOUGH TO DO, KEY TO HEALTH

*T*he cronies are all around the table beginning to eat, when Rodney says, "I want to add one point on mental ability we talked about last week. What about wisdom?

"You go through life gaining experience, and wisdom comes from experience.

"Now Japan bashing irritates me, and we don't need to copy them either, but there is one lesson from Japan I would like to proclaim from ocean to ocean. Charlie sent me this government publication, so let me read . . . 'It doesn't occur to us that some things do get better with time. . . . Some cultures have known this for a long time--the top management of Japanese companies are often men in their 70's and 80's. It is assumed that the wisdom they have acquired is a bonus for their companies. From our perspective at the moment, there's no reason to doubt that.'"

"Tell it to the Ridenhour brothers," says Lear.

Henry finishes his bowl of corn flakes, and Violet fills his coffee cup. "That is a point well taken, Roddy, and is in line with what research has demonstrated. Somehow in this country we've missed that lesson. Old means out, and that is bad policy. Wisdom does count. We can go as long as we desire and are in reasonable health--far longer than generally permitted or admitted."

"Congress, thanks to Claude Pepper, has relaxed the rules on mandatory retirement," says Roddy. "But in retirement or not, it is up to us, personally, each of us individually, to keep going. It is our own view of aging that counts, not society's."

"That's right. The Ridenhour raiders got me out, but they sure didn't get me down."

Henry takes control. "Now, let me mention a good book on the related point, or *Late Life Potential*, by Doctors Kozma and Stones. This is something I have long believed. We have been talking about the maintenance and rejuvenation of the mental condition. Physical performance also declines in older persons because they don't keep in shape. This book cites the evidence. Physical performance and physical condition will improve for older people who take up physical training programs. They say you can even improve your tennis game with overpractice! So it's never too late to start. That's our subject today.

"Now, Joe, Will Mack, Roddy and Victor all have reports. But first let me introduce this distinguished panel by quoting Dr. Robert N. Butler, who is Director of the National Institute on Aging: 'If exercise could be packed into a pill, it would be the single most widely prescribed, and beneficial, medicine in the Nation.'

"So, Joe, you tell us how to concoct the magic exercise pill."

"Nothing to it, Henry. Just roll the stuff together--running or walking, stretching and bending, breathing and puffing, using all muscles--and stuff it in a little capsule marked common sense."

"No," says Lear, "marked will power."

"Whatever. I majored in physical education at State--and baseball--and nobody ever told me exercise gets more important the older you get. It does, though. It wards off heart attacks and stroke. Henry has told us exercise is one guard against cancer, arthritis, and other stuff. Nobody can doubt that exercise is good for you at any age. It is a must for older people"

"But a lot of people overdo it," says Victor Beane.

"Not you. Most of us underdo it," drawls Lear.

"I'll tell you what I do. I walk at least two miles almost every day," says Joe. "It doesn't make any difference if I miss a day or two a week. Some people say every other day is just right. My theory is that if you can get in the habit you can't wait to get out. Until you do, you will come up with all kinds of excuses to wait 'til tomorrow.

"Now you can run if you want to, and I see Lear running some mornings. I don't run very often. I don't like to get exhausted. Your knees get damaged. I do run a little bit during my walks just to prove I can still run.

"I stretch my arms, shoulders, fingers while I'm walking. So, Henry, come to think of it, I do exercise my fingers. First thing every day, rain or shine, I lie on the floor and stretch my arms back, touching the floor with my fingers, and repeat full circles both ways. I then do sit-ups, a dozen, which I think is right for me, but you could do more. Then I roll back, legs straight up, and bicycle, and do scissors, and other motions to limber my hips, knees, legs, ankles, and toes.

"While I'm on the floor I exercise my lower back muscles by exhaling and pressing my lower back against the floor. Sometimes I get so relaxed I want to lie there and take a short nap--but I don't.

"I then do a dozen push-ups, slowly and fully. I then on hands and knees exercise my back and stomach muscles by pushing my stomach with a full breath against my lower back. Then I walk if the weather is right for walking.

"Do I spend too much of my time exercising? No! That's the most useful time of my day." Zaroom slaps both hands on the table.

"Good report, Joe," says Henry. "No question you are in good shape. Now, Will Mack."

"I've been making mental notes on Joe's routine. Sounds good. I want to report on one article, tell one story. They have to do with weight lifting. I used to do twenty pull-ups--chinning--in a flash, and then, suddenly it seemed, I had difficulty doing one. I realized I hadn't tried in years.

"There was a study at Tufts University putting old and frail people through exercises with weights. One old gent who couldn't even get out of his chair without help became able to do so.

"I'll not give you all the details, but the major finding of the study is that a weight-training program will bring dramatic increases in muscles and strength to frail men and women. I didn't know this. People up to 96 years of age were in the program.

"They proved--let me quote them--"that high-intensity strength training is feasible and is associated with significant gains in strength and muscle hypertrophy,'--that means they got bigger--'in individuals up to 96 years of age. However, just as in younger individuals, these changes are not maintained in the absence of continued training.'

And I am sure they didn't mean 96 is the age limit."

"That is good stuff to know," says Roddy.

"Sure, and if it applies to old and frail people, it applies even more to us. Where can we perform these exercises? The YMCA, nautilus or similar equipment, the couple of health clubs in town. I'll talk later about using dumbbells."

"So flabbiness doesn't got to be?" Victor asks. "I've been thinking it just came with age."

"To a degree, it probably does. But we get lazy. We drift into doing less and less. A product of old age can be the frame of mind that I don't have to do anything else I don't want to do. Bad thinking!

"We don't need to get in such bad shape. Weak muscles come from sedentary lifestyle--which we can avoid.

"This report notes in passing that 'muscle strength decreases by perhaps 30 percent to 40 percent during the course of the adult life span.' Their experiment argues that it ain't necessarily so. It seems certain that good physical condition retards the aging process."

"Of course it does," says Joe.

"They do tell us that the gains will be lost if the person quits the strength-building exercises."

"Of course," says Joe.

"Are we ready to go on, Will?" Henry inquires.

"Go on to Rodney, professor. I'll come back with one story."

"Thanks, Will," says Henry. "Roddy, what have you got for us?"

"Well, I had something until you stole my punch line when you told about the exercise pill. Charlie sent me the *Age Page* entitled, 'Don't Take it Easy--Exercise!' This is where your quote came from."

"Sorry 'bout that."

"Never mind. I'll struggle on.

"I've numbered the salient messages: 'One. 'Before starting a fitness program, and most of us haven't, talk to your doctor first.' A phone call will do it.

"Two. 'Regular physical activity can help the human body maintain, repair, and improve itself to an amazing degree.' Remember Norman Cousins insisted that the doctor in the body was his best doctor. Exercise keeps the doctor awake.

"Three. 'Tailor your program. . . . For example, jogging is not for everyone and may be dangerous for those who have unsuspected heart disease.' Joe said he walks.

"Four. Exercise tones your muscles, and helps keep your joints, tendons, and ligaments more flexible."

Five. 'Exercise can strengthen your bones, slowing down the progress of osteoporosis, a bone-thinning disorder common in elderly women.' By all means get your wife involved with you.

"Six. 'Although more research is needed,' the report says, 'there is evidence that exercise may strengthen your heart and lungs, lower your blood pressure, and protect against the start of adult-onset diabetes.' I'd have thought all that was proven. In any event, we already know it's beneficial.

"Seven. 'Exercise may also give you more energy, help you sleep better and feel less tense.' . . .I'm sure it does.

"Finally, they say begin exercising slowly, especially if you have been inactive. Start with short periods of about 5 to 10 minutes twice a week. Then build up slowly.

"I got so carried away that I went at it hard for a couple of days. I could hardly get out of bed this morning."

Henry laughs and says, "Thanks, Roddy. Now Victor, do you have something?"

"I sure do have something and it's my time, boys." Victor Beane unfolds a large printed bulletin. "How come is it that everybody wants to cover up he's walking, like it's something sissy? It takes a whole lot of persistence to walk, but you'll hear people saying, 'Yeah, I jog every morning.' At least Joe brags on his walking, and he is right. Let me read you this: 'Not running, not jogging, but *walking* is not only your most efficient exercise but the only one you can *safely* follow all the years of your life.'

"Lear, you jog?"

"Not really. Only when I see Joe coming."

"Victor, I'm glad we are getting some confirmation," says Will Mack. "I ran, sprinted, jogged, more or less regularly, and then I got wiser and started walking.

"Oh, I looked good jogging in the neighborhood with my 'Central High Bulldogs' sweatshirt. The students loved it. But two of my school friends in the state dropped dead while they were jogging. I figured walking was my game. And you know what I discovered? Walking is mentally therapeutic. I never did much thinking while jogging. I was too occupied panting. Now, walking, I work out my own little problems and most of the world's problems. I think something through, and then I shift subjects. Sometimes I just let my mind wander from 'shoes--and ships--and sealing wax'--to 'cabbages--and kings. . . and whether pigs have wings.'

"All this helps make me anxious to get out and walk--and we need all the little urges that we can get."

Victor slaps the table. "Right on the money, as usual, Mack! I've got this bulletin called 'Executive Health,' which is written by doctors. Walking protects against stress. Walking helps your lungs, your heart and cardiovascular system, weight reduction, and even your bones. Walking uses more than half of your muscles--foot, leg, hips, back. All of this comes from a conference the National Institutes of Health held at Bethesda, and its report says all that and more.

"They tell us what we ought to already know: 'Your body is the one machine that breaks down when it is *not* used. It is the one machine that works *better* the *more* it is used!'

"Now, how far should we walk? They point out that there is not all that much difference in walking and running in terms of calories burned, only twenty percent more in a hard run of six miles than walking the same distance. Of course it takes longer, but it is safer.

The report tells us that 'The advantages you think you get from setting some sort of time record for yourself are far outweighed by the dangers this may impose, particularly as you grow older. Runners and joggers have died from heart attacks by pushing themselves against time.'"

Joe, with a grin, interrupts. "Your mind is slipping, Beanie. You forgot your question. You were going to tell us how far to walk."

"Of course. I'm coming to that. Distance is more important than speed, they tell us. They say, it is the prolonged moderate rhythmic endurance of walking that is so important to your health and long life.

"Now listen to this. Walking is a great way--not a quick and temporary way--to lose weight. You think I haven't been paying attention to this!

"Let me touch on one more. . . ."

"How far?" chirps Joe.

Victor Beane ignores him. "The editors make the point that now walking is being prescribed for those recovering from heart attacks. All of us know that. Jamie, Herb, Helen Blankenship, John Williams, and several others walked in the mall all winter, part of their treatment for their heart rehab.

"Now, here's the nut in the peanut, as Joe says. . . 'if such a program can improve a sick heart, why wait for a heart attack before you start to take care of your heart? *If you are lucky enough to get a second chance!*' Think of that. It's profound, as Will Mack would say.

"Now, Joe, for starters, did you know that the military pace is one hundred and twenty steps a minute?"

"Sure I know it. You know I was a Marine."

"That will take you three and a half miles in an hour. That is good distance for you to walk, if you walk at least five times a week. But you don't necessarily have to walk at that pace. Walking permits you to stop and look at the flowers.

"And here is some more, Joe. After you walk one to three miles at a slow pace for a few weeks, you can pick up the pace and do four miles in an hour. Joe, how far do you walk?

"I'm getting to it," Joe stutters. "Most every day."

"Very good, very good, Beanie!" Henry gives him a little hand-clap.

Rodney Thomas asks, "Henry, may I horn in right here? A friend of mine sent me a little booklet called *Older and Wiser*, a report of the Baltimore Longitudinal Study of Aging. You know that outfit?"

"That's great," Henry answers. "Yes, I looked at their book. Rather formidable. The appendix contains some very good reports of many experiments on many topics."

Roddy opens a little pink booklet. "This ought to be authentic. I'm going to mention some conclusions.

"First, what happens to the aging body? 'The heart grows slightly larger with age. . . . Although the older heart is unable to increase its pumping rate during exercise as much as a younger heart, it appears to compensate by dilating to a greater extent, delivering more blood per heartbeat. . . .'"

Victor interrupts. "What does that prove?"

"It proves something worth knowing. Here is their conclusion: 'The healthy, exercising older heart increases its output in somewhat different but just as efficient manner as the younger heart.'

"That reaffirms for me that we need to keep active, need to keep our muscles in shape, and the old heart will do its part."

Joe Zaroom has recovered. "Right back to activity and exercise!"

"Wait a minute," says Victor, "I'm not through. Here are a few more tips on walking. Build up gradually. Take seriously heart pains, sudden dizziness, cold sweating, fainting.

" On humid days, exercise less and drink lots of water. On cold days, wear less than you would if not exercising, but be warm and wear a cap or hat. Don't exercise too strenuously, and wait about a half hour before gulping down food after exercising. That's it. Walking!"

"I suspect that we just get lazy, say it's too much trouble, I've done all that. It's easier to sit than to sweat," says Rodney.

"Like I say," says Joe, 'It's the best hour of my day."

"Well, professor, if you are ready to dismiss us, I think I'll limp over to the office," Rodney declares.

"Great. I'm going to be out of place for a few days, so I'll see you next Friday. I've got some heavy stuff for you then."

"Now, wait a dad-blimmed minute," says Will Mack. "I haven't even finished my coffee, and besides you owe me one story."

"Sorry 'bout that, Will. I was getting worn out just listening to all the talk about exercising."

"Let me add a little something and then you can go," says Will Mack. "All this walking is okay, but it leaves out for the most part your upper body.

"Joe's exercise gets at all muscles, but I've got another emphasis. Several years ago I told my children, 'Now I have given the world three dumbbells so why don't you give me two for my birthday.' They did. Fifty-pound weights, because they explained that was the weight Timmy could lift, and they figured I was bigger than he. I swapped them for much lighter dumbbells, and each can choose his own proper weight. I use them at least four times a week, and my arms went from being flabby to being right firm today."

"Do you just lift them or is there a science to it?"

"There is a routine. You can get a booklet of exercises with your dumbbells. I use a routine I mostly picked out of a book by Bill Pearl called *Getting Stronger*."

"Well, tell what you do. How long do you work out?"

"You can't work out very long. I lie on my back, knees bent, feet flat, hands by my thighs, and lift the bells at the elbows, then straight up, slowly down at a starting position

"Next, hands stretched from body out. That's tougher. Lift at elbows. Then straight up and slowly down. Be alert not to drop them on your skull. I do one arm at the time, and shield from a slip with the other hand.

"Then I sit in a chair, holding the two weights just beyond my knees, arms along the thighs, then with palms up, use wrists to lower and raise. You can feel the muscles all the way to your shoulders.

"Then, and this is very good, hold only one of the bells, palm up, rest your upper arm against your inner thigh, arm straight, your other hand on your other knee to brace you, and lift weight to your shoulder. Let down slowly and then repeat, and then switch to the other hand.

"That's two lying down, two in a chair, and now two standing.

"Standing, hand hanging dumbbell at your waist, fold at elbow to the shoulders, then push the weight straight up, then slowly down in two movements.

"Last, with one bell held with both hands straight over your head, palms up, lower it behind your head as far as you can and then return."

"Do each of these six movements about ten times, starting with three or four and working up."

"Very interesting," says Rodney. "Can't you use them for your legs and back?"

"I am sure you can, but I don't."

"Sure you can," says Joe. "You do lunges. Hold the dumbbells by your side, erect, and thrust a leg as far forward as you can. Return, and lunge the other leg. There are some movements for your back but I figure that is for the Arnold Swartzbergers."

"Schwartzenager."

"Whatever."

"Glad I waited, Will Mack."

"Now, Henry," says Rodney, "can we struggle to get to our feet and limp out?"

"Exercise," Henry says, "is one of our Final Four. I'll bet it is the hardest one of the requirements we have set for ourselves. I hope we can talk about physical conditioning again. This is one we can accomplish without counting on luck, Joe."

"Why would you say it is so hard?" Joe asks, "nobody is talking about strenuous."

"Takes a lot of will power," says Lear, "and that is what is so hard and gets harder with age. It's so easy to put it off, to cut it short, to put it off 'til tomorrow."

"You're right about that. See you all next Friday. We've got some good stuff on cholesterol. How to get it, and how to get rid of it, and why we have to have it."

They leave a few dollar bills for Violet and flock their way to Gus' s cash register.

Chapter Thirteen

CHOLESTEROL

*H*enry pushes back his cereal bowl, and takes his little notebook out.

"I promised to get some more information about cholesterol, and no question we need to give more than passing attention to cholesterol. I have here the *Report of the Expert Panel on Detection, Evaluation, and Treatment of High Blood Cholesterol in Adults*. It was published by the Public Health Service a couple of years ago."

"What does it mean when you have your cholesterol tested? The first figure you need to look at is your total cholesterol. Your cholesterol count needs to be under 200. If it is 240 it is 'High." In between is borderline."

"Two hundred what?" asks Victor.

"Well, we don't need to know that, but it's milligrams of cholesterol per one-tenth of a liter of blood."

"But we need to know about cholesterol. There is so much about it in the advertisements today. Sounds sometimes like a flimflam"

"Fair enough. First of all, cholesterol is essential to life. It is a fatty substance called a 'lipid' and is a key ingredient in every cell, and the liver normally manufactures what we need and we are constantly eating it or eating what the liver uses to manufacture it.

"In addition to being a part of the cells, it gets there by constantly traveling in the circulating blood, in little protein packages the blood is what is measured, and if it gets too high, this is what we need to worry about."

"Like too much of a good thing," adds Joe Zaroom.

"Sure, we know that cholesterol tends under certain circumstances to attach to the walls of the arteries and clog them up--that is atheriosclerosis--and that is the danger, a principal cause of heart disease and strokes."

"We've already talked about heart disease. Now we are talking about cholesterol and diet. This book tells us that it is one of the three controllable heart attack risk factors we can do something about. The other two are high blood pressure and cigarettes. Right now we need to talk about what we can do to keep our cholesterol levels low."

"Wouldn't you say also that fatness is a controllable risk factor?"

"Yes. I'd say so. Fatness contributes to cholesterol risks."

"Now, Henry, isn't there some good cholesterol?"

"You fellows know more about cholesterol than I do. Sure. If your cholesterol level is high, you should be told how much is the bad kind, LDL, low density lipoproteins. That's what we need to watch, keep it below the 160 level. The good kind is HDL, high density liproproteins. You'd like that to be above 35."

"Okay, we watch it," says Rodney, "and if it gets too high, what do we do about it?"

"The first thing you do is talk to your doctor who tested you. He can suggest several actions, depending on other heart disease risk factors you might have.

"Most likely, he will tell you to restrict certain items in your diet--especially animal fat, stop smoking, and lose fat if you are overweight. He might prescribe a drug, if he thinks your danger is severe enough for that.

"What drugs, what food items?"

"I'll leave the prescription to the doctor since I am not trying to practice medicine, but I can talk about eating habits, right from the book.

"The what to eat is simple, not easy, but simple. Reduce the fat on you, if obese, and reduce the fat you eat, much of which the liver turns into cholesterol. This is the clearest advice. Reduce the amount of fat you eat. The fat you must use in cooking and seasoning should be the non-saturated kind, corn oil or olive oil or some others--read the labels and avoid saturated fats. The new labels tell you.

"Fats are in a bad category of their own, but there are a lot of other foods to watch. The Expert Panel says to cut down--limit not eliminate--foods that contain high cholesterol--eggs, meats, milk, liver, cheese, and by extension all animal products because all contain cholesterol in virtually every cell. The Panel advises that we substitute more fruits, vegetables, breads, cereals, pasta, rice, and beans."

Henry pauses. "Now that is probably not bad advice, for a good diet, but some doubts are now raised whether this kind of diet has much to do with reducing your cholesterol levels. The Expert Panel does report that the cholesterol content of food has an appreciable, but lesser influence than saturated oils, but nevertheless the advice of the Panel is to eat no more than 300 milligrams of cholesterol in foods each day."

"Good Lord! How do we do that? Carry an accountant and a calculator?"

"That would help, but I've made some notes. You can look at food labels, and I can tell you a pound of steak or pork, ten ounces of cheddar cheese, two eggs, or four ounces of beef liver, each has about 300 milligrams of cholesterol."

"That's not too bad," says Victor. "A serving of steak for supper, an egg for breakfast, and a pimento sandwich for lunch."

"Now if you fry that steak in oil, or mix mayonnaise with your pimento cheese, you have crossed the fat line, says Roddy"

"Yeah, but we ought to be able to handle that," says Victor.

"Avoid saturated fats and cut down on cholesterol foods."

"One more important thing," says Henry. The liver uses acetates to manufacture cholesterol. Sugars, including corn sweeteners, especially those in soft drinks are converted in good part to acetates. So sugars are suspect as a big source of excess cholesterol. There hasn't been much research on this, but I am looking for evidence."

"Sugar? That's something new," says Victor.

"More or less new. Dr. William Costelli of the Framingham Heart Study suggests that sugar is harmful only when in a diet of too much saturated fat. Sugar provides the immediate energy, so the fat is stored and comes back to clog the veins. His advice is to avoid excessive sugar. And, as I said, some think sugar is one of the sources of cholesterol.

"Then, some think that cholesterol is not the problem as such. It sticks because it is a relief substance for damage done by unconverted amino acids which scratch and injure the intestine walls. Cooking meats cause the destruction of B-6 which is there to convert the amino acids. I want to investigate this idea."

"You're saying that cholesterol is not the villain, as such."

"I'm saying there needs to be more research. There are some doubts being raised about cholesterol theories. Right now the best advice is to go easy on such foods, and hold animal and other saturated fats to ten percent of your total calories. I would not be surprised to see some new cholesterol theories developed in the near future. Right now, why take chances? Hold down on cholesterol foods and saturated oils, as well as sugars and corn syrups.

"And I have for several years been taking a vitamin B-6 tablet to help convert amino acids."

"I can handle all that," says Victor.

"Now, Victor," says Henry, "let me shift the subject. I have tried to find answers to your question about other heart diseases. As you said, we know that the heart attacks caused mostly by clogged vessels is the big killer, but what about other heart disease?"

"Yes, and what do we do to avoid all of the heart problems?"

"Sure that's a large order. I didn't set out to run a medical school--but I've got together a few comments. Mainly you have to rely on your doctor.

"I can name some of the heart diseases, without daring to say I've named them all. There is arrhythmia, an unreliable heart beat and the ultimate treatment is a pacemaker.

"There are various types of damage to the heart, by infections, or maybe slight birth defects that magnify in time, which reduce its muscle strength, or to the valves, which distort the flow of blood and might get infected by something as trivial as having your teeth cleaned. You must take an antibiotic before dental or surgical work if you have any kind of heart problem from a murmur to a transplant. An infection, if not eliminated, can require a valve replacement, or worse."

"Replace valves inside the heart? Can that be done?"

"It can indeed. Lewis Grizzard had a replacement, a pig valve, said he cried every time he passed a barbecue place. There are, let me add, also synthetic valves. I can't get into all that."

"There is also a condition called deconditioning, meaning loss of strength of the heart muscle and the responsiveness to the central nervous system, thought to result from inactivity."

"Closely related, of course, are the other cardiovascular ailments. For example, phlebitis and the resulting pulmonary emboli, the clots in veins, creating inflammation, and breaking off to trash the lungs. And there are varicose veins, maybe serious, maybe not."

"And Angina. This is not a disease, but a pain which is a result of too little oxygen to the heart wall muscle, which is a result of some artery or related disease. The pain comes on when there is extra exercise or stress, but should last only a few minutes when you stop exercising. See your doctor. He may give you a nitroglycerin tablet for angina."

"I hate to think we face all that. How do we sidestep that stuff?"

"I didn't undertake to practice medicine, so I wouldn't go into all the available treatments, even if I knew. I can tell you two good pieces of news.

"First, medical science has developed successful treatment for most of these disorders.

"Second, and I quote, 'In the absence of disease, cardiovascular performance is capable of remaining excellent throughout life.'"

"So, how do we assure the 'absence of disease'?"

"That's what I need to try to tell you. Your doctor can tell you what to do if you get the disease."

"Tell," says Joe.

"Okay, I'll draw on the advice of the doctor I just quoted: Dr. Robert J. Sullivan, M.D., M.P.H., of Duke University Medical Center. He says quit smoking and keep your blood pressure regulated."

"We already know that."

"Sure you do. Knowing and not doing is our problem. Dr. Sullivan includes some other things we already know. Cut down on fats and sugar and control weight. Control diabetes, or watch for it. Exercise regularly, which he defines as 20 minutes three times a week at 75 percent of your maximum heart rate."

"We ought to exercise more than that," says Joe.

"Except for the word on sugar, that fits our Final Four," says Victor.

"No. We say eat right," Joe declares. "That could cover sugars."

"Whatever," Henry continues. "Let me quote him once more: 'Taken together, such elements comprise a 'healthy life style,' which is being widely promoted in western society. Time will tell the degree to which this effort yields improved health.'"

"Time will tell," Will Mack repeats. "Well, Henry, we can't wait for Time to tell us, so we might as well keep on trying to tell Time."

"I'm with you," says Joe.

"Now Henry, you were also going to talk about some other diseases. Seems to me we can wheel along and protect our heart, brain, and luck out on cancer, and wake up in the hospital with some piddling thing like pneumonia or pink toothbrush which will do us in prematurely like Roddy's log truck."

"Yes, I've thought a lot about that. Should I be looking for an encyclopedia of illnesses? The answer is no. That wasn't my assignment."

"You are right," says Will Mack. We set out to see how we could live longer and better, so we can't expect you to tell us how to get well from every bug that attacks us. Leave it to our doctors.

"Thanks, Will. I can't practice medicine."

"Of course not, Henry, but you did promise to tell how to avoid all these rank-and-file diseases. You can't get off the hook, Henry."

"Now, that's sneaky, Will. But I have been taking a few notes on preventive health care. That is the best general medicine against all bugs."

"I hope you are not going back to the asafetida sack. When I was a kid, some children were still being forced by some old aunt to wear a little sack around the neck in the winter that would repel all germs," Roddy chortles.

"Yea, I remember," laughs Victor. "It repelled everybody. Never smelt anything so foul. They couldn't get close enough to anybody to catch a germ."

"That's about what I've got in mind," says Henry. "Most of us have been avoiding our Final Four program like it was asafetida. The answer is prevention. The older we get, the more preventive action we need.

"Take pneumonia, or most any illness, you try to protect yourself against exposure to raw weather, avoid exhaustion, get regular sleep, and follow the Final Four. The best defense is good health, a healthy lifestyle.

"I have picked out some preventive points. Physical exam, already one of our Final Four Steps, is a preventive tool, and at our age we should go through this every year, and the self-exam every day.

"Dental exams every six months. Eye exams for glaucoma and whatever.

"I'd say take flu shots."

"They're dangerous," says Lear.

"Not really. Not as risky as catching influenza."

"What about pneumonia shots?" Victor asks.

"Ask your doctor."

"Now what else can we take preventive steps against?" Henry asks.

"Drunk drivers," says Roddy.

"Sure, and generally we need to sharpen our defensive driving habits. And look out for log trucks. And fasten your seat belt.

"Hazards in the home?" Henry continues. "Name a few."

"Defective wiring, throw rugs, loose stair rail, icy steps or walks-and--," Roddy chortles, "cheeses and cake in the refrigerator."

"Right! Take an inventory in our own homes. All possible hazards," says Joe.

"And correct them," adds Victor.

"There is one last word," says Will Mack, "if we are talking about preventive care. Nobody can do it for you. Nobody can make you get up and go exercise, as if it were--and it probably is--the most important chore of the day. Nobody is going to eat right as your proxy. You can't hire a hit man to get rid of your pot belly. I believe we fail to grasp the truth that it is up to us personally to slow down aging."

"We get lazy. We've done our watch," says Victor. "Let the ship sail on. We are passengers now--that's the way to slide overboard."

"So, we can make it fun, exciting, to do what we know we ought to be doing," says Will Mack. "Can we get up in the morning as anxious to go exercise as we are to read the sports page? Can we follow the Final Four like it was our life's work?"

"I don't know," says Roddy. "But I think that's what we've been telling each other."

You've got it," Henry nods. "We pretty well know how to keep in shape. We really know how to grow old. We just don't know how to make ourselves follow our own advice."

"Just kick your own rear end when you start goldbricking," says Joe.

"Time to go," announces Roddy.

"See you next Friday."

"Well, Henry," Will Mack laughs, "you sidestepped and straight-armed my question about rank and file disease. But you crossed the goal for a touchdown, anyhow. We avoid, as best we can, all disease by preventive care, basically our Final Four."

"And luck," adds Joe.

"Right you are, both of you, and thanks. See you next Friday. Roddy will report on a lesson his secretary taught him."

"That'll be an upgrade."

Chapter Fourteen

BEHOLD THE PYRAMID.
EAT FAT, GET FAT

Henry hasn't finished his food, but he pounds the table for attention. "Roddy has read what I think is an interesting book. Are you Roddy ready--ready, Roddy?"

"Sure, I always have my homework."

"Now, I am not going to vouch for this but it is worth considering. I never trusted these diets of meat only, carbohydrates only, nothing but bananas, grapefruit, and the like. I just counted calories but I never had much luck. I could lose eight or ten pounds, and then somehow I wearied of well doing. And went back up.

"My secretary kept bugging me about a low fat diet. I told her I knew fat was heavy with calories, had to be counted, and that anyhow I used only unsaturated oils and margarine. No difference, she said, all fat is likely to end up on your waistline.

"I kept explaining to her that she didn't understand so she bought me a book. I am going to tell you what it says. It is a paperback book and I don't trust paperback books about diets. Anyhow I read it.

"Here is the book's theme. 'You can't get fat except by eating fat.'" Roddy nods as if he has completed his speech.

"That's all?" asks Will Mack.

"Just about. I have already lost 7 pounds."

"The heck you say. But you have lost 7 pounds before. What's different?"

"Well, this time I didn't count calories. I just counted fat grams."

"For heaven's sake tell us more. Is there anything to this diet?"

"Actually it's a right good book. I'm glad I own it. But I'm not recommending its diet. That's up to you. I'll tell you about it, I suppose.

"Fats, carbohydrates and proteins burn calories and supply energy differently. Protein, in any ordinary diet, doesn't put on fat. It takes a fourth of the energy in protein just to convert it for the body's use. Surplus carbohydrates, they've learned, do not convert easily to body fat--only about four percent on a normal day.

"Any surplus fat eaten and not burned goes almost directly to body fat, 97 percent efficient. The other side of the coin is that the body must have fat in the mix to produce energy, so if it doesn't get enough dietary fat, it will withdraw the needed amount from the body's stored fat. That's the story." Roddy sits back.

"Dammit, don't make us beg," says Lear. "Tell us more."

"So count only fat grams--eat as little as 30 to 60 grams of fat a day, depending on what energy you are burning."

"Don't you think this is just another quack idea to sell a diet book?" Will Mack insists.

"It might be. But I think the chances are that it is not. It was developed at Vanderbilt University, the Vanderbilt Weight Management Program. That gives any proposition a lot of credibility. The director of that program and the author of this book, a Vanderbilt professor of psychology, is almost sure to be on the up and up. In addition this idea has a ring of common sense about it."

"I'll buy that," Murphy interrupts, "but I don't want to clear all professors of psychology."

"You were one of them, weren't you," Joe sniggers.

"Well, not quite, but almost, so I know them."

"You fellows get serious. There is a ring of common sense," Roddy continues. "Let me read from page one: 'All calories are not the same to the human body. When it comes to being overly fat or overweight, it's primarily the fat calories that count, *not* the carbohydrate and protein calories.'

"And from page three: 'A hundred calories of baked potatoes and 100 calories of French fries are not equal, except in the laboratory! . . . Indeed, the differences in the way your body metabolizes fat compared with protein and carbohydrate are so great that . . . you can't get fat except by eating fat!' That is the story. You can read the book for the details."

"I'll have to say that sounds sensible," says Vic Beane.

"Dr. Martin Katahn, who wrote the book, based his opinions on recent studies, and he tried it out and proved it on people.

"You can try it if you want to. I'll loan you my copy. Let me leave two thoughts with you. To lose weight, holding to 30 grams of fat a day is a good target. That's what I'm doing. A gram of fat is 9 calories, and a tablespoon of oil--any kind--contains 14 grams of fat and 120 calories. Twice that is about the fat grams you can use in a day if you are going to work off that inner tube around your waist and wherever else your body stores excess fat."

"That doesn't give us much margin, does it?" comments Victor. "It takes that much to fry a couple of fish."

"Right, about thirty fat grams from all sources. But you can be fairly free about eating anything else if you keep your fats total down--and it ain't easy. That's the book."

"Let me put you a question," says Will Mack. "If I eat a pile of baked potatoes, macaroni, beans, bread, jello, all carbohydrates, say three thousand or more in a day, could I lose weight? Does the body not get enough energy without the fat so that no fat would be withdrawn from the body, no weight lost--maybe gain a little?"

"That is a good question--but a sorry diet--but the answer is that if you eat zero fat, you will lose weight, and they proved it at Vanderbilt in a thing they call a 'calorimetry chamber.' The fuel mixture required by the body requires fat. Not enough fat in the diet means that fat is withdrawn for the fat storage in the body.

"You can't get fat if you don't eat fat. But I'm not saying gorge yourself on everything else, and neither is Vanderbilt. Excess carbohydrates do convert to fat.

"Carbohydrates are initially stored differently. Let me follow my notes. Converted first to glucose, which the cells burn for energy, excess carbohydrates are stored in the liver and in the muscles as glycogen where it can be quickly retrieved and transformed back to glucose for immediate use when needed. It takes eight times as much energy to convert excess carbohydrates to body fat as it takes to turn dietary fat to body fat."

Will Mack continues. "But you could gain weight if you didn't eat anything but pure carbohydrates and protein, surely?"

"Not so."

"That just doesn't seem to be right. Food is food and food is energy!"

"That's what I always thought--I'm trying to find an illustration--here it is: From page 15--'Even if you take in a large amount of carbohydrate, practically none of it will be turned into fat. In fact, in one of the studies . . . the research subjects ate a single meal containing 2000 carbohydrate calories. Only 81 of those calories were turned to fat, and, because the body burns a mixture of fat and carbohydrate for fuel, the subjects had to burn stored body fat in the hours that followed that meal.

In other words, in spite of consuming 2000 carbohydrate calories in a single sitting, they began to lose body fat!'"

"Wow!" says Joe.

"But no one suggests that one-time experiment as a regular diet , and their guinea pigs were probably young students."

"Okay," says Vic Beane. "How do we count grams? What do we have to give up?"

"This is a 300-page book, and much of it is taken up with recipes and a fat index. Avoid oils. Read labels, and look for grams of fat. Hold to two tablespoons--18 grams, 240 calories-- if you want to lose weight. Dr. Kathan said he had found that his chief culprits were cheese and mayonnaise."

"Add peanut butter and you've made the case against me," says Victor Beane.

"Henry," asks Will Mack, "You said last week that we shouldn't let more than 30 percent of our calories be fat. In a mere 1500 calorie diet, that would be 450 calories."

"Sure, no conflict," says Roddy. "Murphy was talking about a maintenance diet. Today we are talking about a weight-reduction diet. I'm trying to dig into my spare tire. You and Joe are trying to maintain your good weight. Now here are some tips from Dr. Katahn.

"He says use low fat milk. Eat sherbet instead of ice cream. Trim meats and take skin off the chicken. Broil fish. Can't fry anything-- or at least not so often, not while you're trying to lose. One good order of French fried potatoes gives you most of your 30 grams, and a double beef cheeseburger gives you twice your daily quota. That one quick order is about a three-day quota of fat.

"Eat all the fruit, vegetables, cereals, legumes that you want. If you are eating candy, Vic, remember a small chocolate bar has more fat grams than a tablespoon of lard. The book gives you all this information."

"Well, I'll be. Don't fret about calories, but hold down the fat until you've lost all the fat you want to lose. I believe I can live with that." Victor reaches for the book.

"Roddy, that is a good report. Very interesting. I never thought about the difference in the way the body burns calories."

"Well, Murph, I said I don't vouch for it. But it is working for me, and it seems to me to make a lot of sense." Roddy has passed the book to Lear who is examining it.

"Shows you can learn a lot from your secretary."

"If you've got sense enough to listen."

"Now," Henry begins, "is a good time to talk about diet. I'm not talking about going on diets. Roddy was talking about cutting down fats, not dieting as such. I'm really talking about nutrition."

"I'll skip most of the business of fats because Roddy talked about them. You can write it down. All experts agree that most of us eat too much fat."

"Now Rodney didn't have much to say about proteins. I learned from this Columbia University article that we must have the amino acids produced by protein. And the National Institute on Aging tells us that protein 'enables growth and repair of body cells and helps the body resist disease by forming antibodies.' "And they remind us, protein is the basic material in all cells of our body. Columbia suggests that about fifteen percent of our calories should come from proteins--red meats, eggs, poultry, pork, fish-- and legumes, nuts, and grains."

"Why just fifteen percent?" asks Roddy.

"One thing, to get more fiber and energy-producing carbohydrates."

"We need protein in every cell, don't we?" asks Victor.

"Sure," Henry explains, "but too much frequently brings too much fat, keeps us from essential carbohydrates, is bad on the kidneys, and may add to cholesterol problems."

"Well, I reckon that is a good answer."

"I think so. Now if we accept those figures, over half of our calories should come from the carbohydrates. That should be easy to keep in mind--less than a third from fats (and fats calories count up fast), about half that much in calories from meats and other proteins. You are not going to measure everything, but you can keep this pattern in mind."

"The new U.S. food pyramid shows those proportions."

"And," says Roddy, "remember the underlying rule: Don't eat too much."

"Remember old Cornaro, one little thrush per week."

"Okay, Henry, what about vitamins and minerals?"

I'll get to that soon. I have just received a copy of 'the authority.' And I'm working on it. I also have two other good books.

"We've got a little time left. Victor, I believe you had an exercise book your son sent you."

"Henry, we've talked a lot about exercise. So I don't have to tell the guys about this book."

"Not at all. Go ahead. Exercise may be our most important subject."

"First it tells you just what effect exercise has on all aspects of the body--what it does for you--and what the lack of it does to you."

"We already know it's good for us." says Joe Zaroom.

"Did you know that twenty minutes of good walking is better for reducing tension than any drug?"

"Sure it is. Everybody knows that," says Joe.

"Maybe, but I didn't, and this is from an expert. Do you know, Joe, that there is a scientific reason for this?"

"Bound to be."

"Well, everybody doesn't know that, Joe. Like taking tranquilizers, walking lowers the electrical activity in the muscles. But let me tell you some other things about exercise."

"What's the name of the book, Vic?" asks Will.

"Oh. *The Body and Exercise,* by Dr. Morton Bogdonoff who was in the Duke Longitudinal Studies. It gives reasons why exercise is so necessary. Very easy to read, Joe. You could handle it."

"I could write it!"

"I know you could. Did you know that in their tests they showed that older people who have continued exercise have reaction times faster than non-exercisers thirty or forty years younger?"

"I don't doubt it."

"Well, if all that is so, why don't more people exercise?" asks Rodney.

"More people are exercising. Our question is why do so many older people quit exercising?" says Henry.

"I'm one of them," says Rodney. "I've started exercising and quit--more times than Beanie's started diets and more times than Lear has quit smoking--it's hard to bring yourself to do it."

"Hard or not, exercise does so many things for us. Read this book. Exercise gets rid of depression, puts you in a happier mood-- directly affects the central nervous system.

"We've already gone into what it does for our muscles. And the lungs--their health and capacity. To test your lungs, he says, if you take a deep breath and can hold it 45 seconds or more, your lungs are working all right. If you can't, exercise will build back your lung power."

"Can you hold your breath that long?" asks Joe Zaroom.

"Sure can. Tried it last night when I read this. Can you?"

"Well, let's all see who can hold his breath the longest," demands Joe.

"For heaven's sake, Joe, we'll try it at home," says Rodney. "The other customers already think we are nutty. Go on Vic."

"Joe, you hold your breath until I finish this sentence."

"Sure I can."

"Exercise activates the endocrine/hormone system, sending hormones and needed chemicals to all parts of the body," Victor is reading very deliberately, "'assuring among other things that blood clots will dissolve more quickly, that insulin will better regulate sugar...

"'...and the pituitary gland activity is increased', and that is connected with your brain, Joe, 'and the adrenal gland responds better in producing crucial steroids, and favorably affects the maintenance of needed salt and water...

"'...and exercise has a beneficial effect on mental health and disperses anger and aggressive feelings, and while it is more obvious that exercise benefits muscles and the cardiovascular system and the respiratory system...

"'...the doctor points out that exercise is needed by the brain and all the systems, endocrine and nervous, and all of the interlocking mechanisms that keep us going and healthy, and puts your joints and bones in better shape, and that no other. . . .'"

"Whew," Joe explodes. "That was more than 45 seconds.'"

"'. . . no other single action will contribute so much to our well-being as will exercise.'

"You did pretty well, Joe."

"Yeah, but my pituitary gland shut down my brain. You mind going through that once more?"

"You're all right, Joe! Now this book gives a lot of information I am not going into. Good book to have at home. I did pick out a few more points, if you don't mind, Henry."

"No, no, Vic. Go right ahead."

"Okay. Some exercise programs in books are so gung ho that they discourage older people like us. Most of us have not kept up the habit of systematic exercise, but we can build back up more than we think. He says if your exercise for the past ten years has been watching TV it will take you ten months to get back to your previous condition."

"The good news is that you can build back," says Rodney.

"Right."

"Did he say anything about how much?" asks Will Mack. "I've noticed that people who go at it like they were training for a gold medal usually don't last very long."

"Yes, he said don't overdo it, that more is not always better, that the exercised body needs time to recover and develop."

"Weight lifters know this," says Joe. 'They have to wait a day or so for muscle growth to catch up."

"He also said, Will, no less than three times a week, and exercise that amounts to something, gets you sweating and panting at least a little, and he says slow down if you get stitches in your side or feel too fatigued, or dizzy or short of breath. Don't get ahead of your supply of oxygen.

"Oh, yes, and in his book he lays out exercise schedules and programs, if you want to see them."

"Now," says Will Mack, "we have talked about walking, about muscle building, and about exercising our joints. Does he tell us something about back problems? I've always thought that we were ruining our backs without knowing it."

"Yes, I've got it right here. If you have a slipped or herniated disc, you've got a problem for your doctor, so let me skip that.

"Most people have back problems because of poor muscle tone, he says."

"I think that's right. We sit too much. We slump too much. I hassled my students for years. Sit up straight! Your spine is the super highway of the nervous system, everything hangs on it."

Victor sorts through several papers in his hand. "I wasn't going to bore you with the details--but I made notes for myself because my back is always going out. You might guess that back trouble could relate to the bones, the discs--tissue between the vertebrae-- the nerves that might be pinched, damaged, or diseased. I'll leave those back troubles to your doctor.

"There are muscles surrounding the spine--lots of them--to the arms and shoulders, to the rib cage, to the neck and skull. The ones most likely to give us trouble are those in the lower back, those related to the pelvis, to the stomach muscles, to the hips and thighs.

"He did say that most back complaints relate to the lower back, most likely to be the muscles. Like spraining an ankle, you can sprain your back--by picking up something the wrong way, by tension and stress, or twisting the wrong way, or even by sneezing. If the stomach muscles are weaker or stronger than the lower back muscles, things get out of balance. A pot belly is a sign of weak stomach muscles, he says."

"Sounds mighty personal," Rodney laughs.

"You and me are working on it. Here's what happens. To sound like Henry, let me use the word 'lumbosacral' for lower back, and tell you that when there is a strain or sprain or jarring, and your muscles are not strong enough to resist, your lower back muscles go into spasm and that causes more spasm and pain, and the muscles tighten up, and sometimes the back is almost too stiff to move even if you could stand the pain of moving, and sometimes the pain radiates into the buttocks and thighs and down the legs, and this is called sciatica because the sciatic nerve is carrying all this pain down even to your toes."

"Give me the scientific explanation," says Joe.

"You don't think I can. When muscles contract or cramp they use up the oxygen and nutrients, the blood vessels constrict and limit supply, and the waste is not carried off from the cells, and this trouble activates the nerve fibers and the pain is felt and feeds on itself and gets worse. Even when the spasm stops, the pain continues until the supply and waste disposal get back in balance."

"That's right," says Joe. "When you get a charley horse, and walk it off, you can still feel the pain for a long time."

"Thank you, Doctor Zaroom" Victor continues. Now for the treatment. Heat and bed rest, he says, and 'possibly some medication to relax the muscles and relieve the pain.'"

"Let me interrupt," says Lear. "I'd say to take the muscle relaxant medicine right away. I've had a lot of experience with this. You don't even need a prescription. It is in the pain-killer section. Your druggist can tell you. The kind I get has a bolt of lightening on it. As I understand it, the muscle spasms cause more spasms so the thing to do is to relax the muscles."

"And leg cramps can be stopped by quinine," adds Joe. "'Specially those that come in the night. You can buy little pills."

"Or drink gin and tonic," says Rodney.

"Well and good," says Lear, "but get me back to the back. We've got the treatment about right, but what did he say about prevention of back problems? Exercise?"

"You got it right, exercise is the best preventive, so says the doctor. Walk erect, and exercise your back muscles. The book shows sit-ups, leg raises, lying flat and pulling your knees to chin. Another exercise is to lie flat and raise your pelvis.

"He doesn't mention the stomach and back presses that Zaroom told us about, but he does remind us of the upper back muscles. Shoulders back, standing, inhale as much as possible, hold for a count of five, exhale slowly.

"Stand with arms extended straight out, move them to one side, then to front, alternate with palms up and down. Arms straight up, palms touching, slowly down to each side parallel with floor, return to overhead.

"Standing straight, move your head back as far as possible, hold for count of five, return to normal. Hands clasped behind head, elbows back, twist body slowly to right, then return, then to left, then return.

Victor pauses. "I'd say, do each of these ten times."

"I'm going to add those to my exercises," says Joe.

"That might get to the shoulder muscles, and even the joints?"

"And the neck. But I've said what I intended to say. The book lays out a "Forever Fit" program, and some of you might want to follow it. One thing--should we cut back on exercise as we grow older? His answer-- 'Age is not a limitation.' And that's it, Henry."

"'Age is not a limitation!' I like that," says Joe.

"Thank you, Will. That was great."

"Now we have had four lessons today," says Henry. Fat puts on fat. Calories should be about half carbohydrates, one-third or less fat, half that much protein. Exercise has more good side effects than we might have guessed, and is absolutely essential. Back problems can be handled sometimes. We've done a good day's work.

"I'm working on the books about vitamins, and a little more about what I believe is exciting, antioxidants."

"Sounds good," says Roddy. "Let's go earn a living."

Chapter Fifteen

DANGER SIGNS OF AGING

*H*enry has taken out his little notebook, and Violet has taken the orders.

"Well guys," Violet shakes her head. "You are starving your-selves to death, and you're going to starve me too. I think tips should be based on how long you stay, not how much you eat."

"We'll take it up with the committee," drawls Lear.

"I'll be back with your birdfeed." Violet leaves shaking her head.

Henry takes out his little notebook. "I have a couple of books to bring to your attention."

"Joe, haven't we agreed that for older people physical exercise is essential?"

"Sure we have. You'll wither away if you don't exercise."

"I think we all agree, so let me give you a quick review of an-other book that has some useful lessons for us. The title is *Biomark-ers* and it is written by three researchers from Tufts University. Then I have another book on aging, which fits in with the concept of biomarkers."

"The book is based on a study of people in their 70s, 80s, and 90s. Turned out they could do more physically than the researchers guessed they could.

"Here are two points from their introduction, one that we probably did not know.

"First, exercise can make you stronger at any age. We've already heard that muscles can be built at any age.

"Second, bed rest is most likely harmful for older people, even for 'the sick and frail.'"

"That's absolutely true. I've seen people take to the bed and just waste away," says Lear.

"It's soft in the head to stay in the bed," chirps Joe.

"Fair enough, Joe. Now, there are biomarkers--physical functions that decline with age--about which we can do something to retard or reverse."

"Sounds good, Henry," says Joe. "How many?"

"I'll mention just several, Joe Boy. This word doesn't have too precise a definition. Could be a marker of gray hair, deafness, wrinkles, or the need for stronger reading glasses, but those are not the biomarkers these researchers are talking about. Let me proceed.

"First, Roddy, you'll like this. They give us a new word: 'sarcopenia.' It means a body that has turned to fat and flab, too weak to be self-sufficient. This book tells us how to avoid that 'disease.' You'll like it--the new word, that is.

"I like the word better than my sarcopenia--but I'm working on it."

"First let me talk about biomarkers of muscle mass and strength.

"Just losing weight is the wrong way to look at the problem. Roddy, I like your fat makes fat report, but we need more muscle as well as less fat. Your rate of metabolism--using food-- will be higher, and your general health will be better. The objective is to add muscle."

"That makes sense. We talked about getting rid of fat. Can you diet yourself to muscle?"

"Ha! You have to work. But we know you can build muscle, even now."

"We've already heard that."

"Proven fact. It is worth repeating. May be the most important lesson to remember: As you get older, the lurking villain is a sedentary life."

"Agreed," says Rodney, "but some loss of strength is unavoidable?"

"Maybe, but the book says ' . . . we can make a bold assertion: A decline in muscle strength and size is not inevitable.'"

"Hard to believe."

"But it is based on research."

"Say it is just almost true."

"Fair enough."

"Yes, we can stop a decline in muscle strength, but can we actually build back new muscles?" asks Victor.

"A proven fact! You and I can gain muscle right now, and they tell us how."

"So you tell us."

"Exercise. You know that! The point is--that you may not have believed--is that exercise will build back muscle strength at any age."

"Worth getting up for breakfast just to hear that," says Victor.

"It is good news," Henry proceeds, "but first let me tell all of you these researchers say losing weight is the wrong goal. You should more or less forget about your weight. Instead, shed fat, gain muscle."

"Totally reasonable," says Rodney. "My book preached losing fat by not eating fat. Gain muscle by exercise. Keep going, Henry."

"And muscles mean health," says Joe.

"As I said," Henry goes on, "that is the toughest advice to follow. And I believe, the most important. Now let me talk about the second biomarker, your aerobic capacity--how well you can pump oxygen to your muscles."

"You talking about aerobic dancing?"

"No. That too, but walking is aerobic--when we get our pulse up, and sweat good, and breathe hard. That's aerobic, conditioning the heart and lungs to get oxygen to the muscles more efficiently. Helps endurance. Keeps you so you can climb steps. Burns excess fat. Strengthens your arteries and heart. Builds muscles."

"We already have made exercise one of the Final Four."

"Right. Now the amount of cholesterol, you might guess, is another biomarker. Knock off saturated fats to lower the harmful LDL cholesterol. You should exercise, lose body fat, which will raise the level of HDL, the good kind.

"And there is one more thing you'll like. They say a small amount of alcohol will increase HDL, the good cholesterol--but they seemed reluctant to trust us with that information."

"I'll tell my preacher."

"The fourth biomarker is blood pressure. We have already learned a lot about that. The lesson is, don't monkey with blood pressure. Keep it tested and do something about it. High blood pressure will kill you."

"We've already talked about that."

"Sure, and don't forget it." Henry sounds like a first sergeant.

"Biomarkers? That just a fancy word for signs of aging?"

"Fair enough definition. The danger signs!

"But let me summarize. You can, and you better, get your blood pressure and cholesterol tested, and lose fat, and exercise for aerobic capacity and to build muscles."

"Fits the Final Four," says Joe.

"Sure, and I think another book fits here, with exercise and muscles and strength. It's called *The Aging Skeleton*, by a man who obviously enjoyed his work. Are you shorter now than when you were thirty, Joe?" Henry asks.

"I 'spect so. Never was very tall."

"Dr. Spencer L. Rogers tell us the bones age, and may shrink slightly in size, and people become somewhat shorter, but such loss of height is likely to be because of posture, and aging posture is caused by decreased elasticity of the cartilages which certainly we can't do much about, and muscle tone, which maybe we can do a lot about. "Neck muscles need to be kept strong, as do back muscles. The good doctor speaks of the 'inevitable stoop during older years' as causing height reduction, but we might want to take issue with the word 'inevitable.'

"Back pain, he says, may be the result of disk deterioration and rupture, which in turn squeezes the spinal nerve roots. We've talked about that. When the disks loose their elasticity the muscles tend to restrict motion by acting as a brace, which may lead to spasms, which increase disk pressure and you are the victim of a cycle. Bed rest relieves the pressure but he tells us also that bed rest could tend to atrophy the muscle."

"Right. And we already know to keep out of bed."

"Especially somebody else's."

"Stay on the subject, Joe."

"Now," says Henry, "keeping your skeleton healthy depends largely on activity. So it's not just your muscles you are working on--but your bones."

"Exercise helps bones and joints," says Joe. "We know that."

"You know it, and now we know it. Dr. Rogers assures us that the bone system is typically efficient, 'has remarkable strength and powers of self-repair,' and absent dire disease and accident 'usually works well as age advances, with little cause for alarm on the part of its possessor.' He also wryly notes our bones may outlast us by centuries. Some thought!"

"What else?" asks Joe. "We've talked about loss of calcium."

"That's about it, Joe Boy. All of these biomarkers tell how we are aging, all can be starting points for improving our health, and your nut in the peanut is that it is never too late to start improving your health."

"And that," says Roddy, "is what we have been saying since we started all this study."

"There are good books. These researchers are missionaries for strength, for muscle building, and they are completely convincing that muscles can be built back at any age, from almost any poor condition."

"Good going," says Victor. "To me it is exciting that I can build muscles at my age. I can feel my muscles getting tighter just thinking about it."

"Sure can. And we can't talk enough about the need to exercise," Henry puts his little notebook into his shirt pocket."

"What's next?" asks Joe.

Rodney raises his hand. "Hold long enough for me to tell you about this Senate Committee report on lifelong learning. The theme is that the aging society is not aging as much as they think. At 65 most people are not ready to hang it up. They are not worn out. They are not ready to die.

"Some want to retire when they can, and others love their work and want to keep on their jobs, or to work at other things if they are required to retire. So hear this: 'The potential for growth, development, and creativity exists throughout life.'

"The report goes on, 'In our time-starved society, where there is never enough time to do everything we want to do, increased longevity is a gift beyond all expectations."

"Beyond all expectations! I'm glad you mentioned that," says Victor. "I need to tell you that I have signed up for violin lessons. Always wanted to play the violin, bought one from the pawn shop, had it fixed up, and have been to my first two lessons."

"Good gosh," says Joe. "You can't get your fingers to fit on those little strings."

"You better believe I can. Mrs. Kitchen says it will probably help my arthritis. Said if she could teach a four-year old, she could sure teach me. And even if I don't get to Carnegie Hall, I'm doing something I always wanted to do."

"That's great, Beanie. Do you know who invented the violin?"

"Well no, Will Mack, I don't suppose I do. As I said, I got mine from the pawn shop."

"You might surprise Mrs. Kitchen by dropping the fact that the violin was invented in Cremona, Italy, which became the center of violin making.

"One Gasparo Bertolotti invented it in the 16th century, and the brothers Amati claimed to have perfected it."

"I bet Mrs. Kitchen already knows that."

"Now wait a dadgummed minute," says Joe. "This is a setup. How do you know that? Hear it on Jeopardy?"

"As a matter of fact, Joe, you are in the company of an eminent scholar. Since we are all confessing, I've got me a study project, Beanie. I decided I was going to read history. Ancient history--I've lived through modern history. I'm working on four books right now, read most every night, shift from one to the other, and last night just happened to be reading a history of music."

"Terrific! You are both making my point," says Rodney. "Let me get back to the Senate book. Got a lot of suggestions.

"Colleges in most states give older people a break on tuition. Some have special programs for older people, and some have older people teaching special classes. So there are all kinds of ways to go back to school. Check 'em out.

"I've been thinking about going out to the Community College to take auto repair. It's been a long time since I knew all there was to know about a Model T Ford, and besides I've got a 1964 Oldsmobile convertible I want to rebuild. But let me proceed.

"There is something for everybody, really is something for every older person. There are lots of informal study programs. The booklet lists so many. Know somebody who never learned to read? They can do it now. The union has a program at their union hall, down on Caldwell Street. Night school at Grainger High will give people at long last a chance to get their high school diploma.

"Want to study all over the world? Gold mining in Australia, jungle ecology in Brazil, Alexander the Great in Greece, marine science in Bermuda, courses for several weeks, sponsored by Elderhostel if you are 60 years or older, so write them in Boston at 75 Federal Street.

"One college teaches senior citizens social needs of the area, and then provides volunteer opportunities to do something about improving the communities in the region.

"You can get into writing poetry, making pottery, painting pictures.

"There are 9,000 senior centers serving 8 million citizens across the country, so at least 9,000 varieties of local programs. And don't forget the libraries. Not only books, tapes, videos but most of them have a running series of programs. Ours does, and I know we all catch those speakers from time to time.

"Henry, I've hit the highlights. This is one book you can get free, and there's lots more in it. I got mine from Congressman Rose."

"Okay, Rodney! That's a terrific lesson," says Victor. "Never quit--the world is full of new things."

"Very good," says Henry. It's time to go, I suppose. Will, you're going to have your report on your feisty friend?."

"Who is that?" asks Joe.

"I'll let you know. I might not have my report ready."

"See you Tuesday."

Chapter Sixteen

VITAMIN SUPPLEMENTS --
TO TAKE OR NOT TO TAKE?

*V*iolet came to pour coffee, having already removed the dirty dishes. "You sure got out of here in a hurry last time. I was afraid you'd forgot the tips."

It would pay us to put you on a salary," says Lear.

"I'm not complaining, just talking."

"Stay on the cheapskates, Violet," says Henry. "Now, let's talk about vitamins.

"I have just managed to get this official book on vitamins. It is published by the National Academy of Science, and is the 10th edition of *Recommended Dietary Allowances*. I am going to tell you what they say you need and don't need. Then we'll argue about the big question: How to get the vitamins?"

"Before you get in too deep," says Rodney Thomas, "you know my doctor has been saying vitamin tablets are a waste of money. Americans have the most expensive urine in the world, with all those needless vitamins just washing through."

Lear sits up straight and snaps at Roddy. "What's the big deal about costly pee?" You might say the same thing about bath water! All that extra soap makes American bath water the most expensive going into sewers. If vitamins are washing through, that shows we are getting enough. If none is washing through, we are missing what we ought to have. Taking vitamins is good insurance. Shows we are not getting short-changed on what we need. Let some wash through. It proves our point!"

"Lear, you ought to be a tent preacher," Roddy laughs.

"Well, I'll let you both decide that after I tell you what I have found out about vitamins. This is the report that sets the "U.S. RDA"--recommended daily allowance--you see on food labels. "First, you know there is a lot of misinformation about vitamins and nutrients. So much commercial promotion, so many and various claims. All of this breeds either over-reliance or skepticism.

"This book, right or wrong, is the supreme authority in the United States, the last word, on nutrients for healthy people. Says so on the cover. A formidable array of scientists and specialists from several organizations participated in its conclusions. All of this work was done under the umbrella of the National Academy of Sciences, which was granted a charter by Congress in 1863. So this is no paperback publication."

"Fair enough," muttered Lear, "as you like to say, Henry. But for myself, I say it may be the word but not necessarily the gospel. I don't know that I trust the RDA people."

"Okay, fair enough. But let me give you the essence of the book. There is some comment about the need for older adults, those over fifty."

"Well, why fifty?" asks Joe Zaroom.

Lear sits up straight again. "I can tell you that is one more piece of evidence that this crowd is living in the past. Fifty is middle age. If they want to put older people in a category, they ought to start no lower than 65. Those in the sixties are the youngsters of older America."

"Maybe. I wish we had been having these conversations when we were forty. There is an indication in the book that the scientists believe there should be different recommendations for seventy-plus, but there is not presently enough data, they say."

"That's the trouble with RDA," Lear continues. "Not enough research."

"The point is that--I'll read it here--'. . . increasing age may alter nutritional requirement due to change in lean body mass, physical activity, and intestinal absorption. . . . For example, intestinal absorption, particularly of minerals, may be impaired.'"

"So," says Lear, "We need to take in a little more of vitamins to make up for slow absorption?"

"I'd surely think so," answers Henry, "but these experts say there is 'no evidence that an increased intake . . . is necessary.'"

"No evidence the other way, either," Lear growls. "They don't need more evidence. It's common sense."

"I agree, don't blame me."

Rodney speaks up, "You're talking about 'taking more,' meaning you are thinking in terms of pills. Don't they say we should get all these nutrients from a balanced diet?"

"Of course we should. Do you?"

"No, I'm sure I don't. But shouldn't we be talking about balanced diets instead of vitamin pills?"

"Rodney, the damned doctors are all against vitamin tablets. I don't believe anything is taught about vitamins in medical schools," Lear snorts.

"I'll go to the book," Henry says quietly. "'. . . the subcommittee recommends that diets should be composed of a variety of foods that are derived from diverse food groups rather than by supplementation. . . .'"

"There they go again. Always talking about a balanced diet. They think everybody is a trained nutritionist. I bet not two of you know what they meant by 'diverse food groups,'" Lear insists.

"Meats, vegetables, fruit, cereals," snaps Joe Zaroom.

Vic Beane adds, "Fats, carbohydrates, proteins. . . ."

"There you are!" says Lear. "There's no way people are going to figure all of that out every day. No reason to. No way to know whether you are short some valuable vitamin. What is the big deal about taking vitamin tablets every day? Cost too much?"

"There are a lot of hucksters in the business. It is the modern snake oil, the modern medicine show," says Rodney.

"There are hucksters in the insurance business, too, Rodney, but you are legitimate," says Will Mack. "There are legitimate vitamin tablets. It's like insurance, too. I hope I don't need fire insurance, but I buy it just in case I do. I hope I get all the vitamins I need from Gus, at home, at the hot dog stand, and the American Legion hut, but just in case I don't, I take vitamins every morning and every night. It is good insurance in case I missed the balanced diet somehow. If it all washes out, so be it.

"I'll sure buy that," snaps Lear.

"Now Rodney, I bet you can find that your corn flakes, your milk, your margarine, and a number of other foods have been fortified. What is the difference in that and taking vitamin tablets?"

"You fellows want to start an argument? I was just telling you what the doctor said, and Henry read the same thing from the book."

"Yes, but they are wrong. They are blind and don't want to see," Lear declares.

"Okay," Henry interrupts. "Let's talk about the main vitamins, and we can vote later on how to get them.

"Vitamin A helps vision, growth, cell reproduction, and protects the immune system. This is right from the book."

"Let's hear it for vitamin A," claps Joe Zaroom.

Henry continues. "Vitamin A comes from liver and fish liver oils, from whole milk and eggs, and from carrots and spinach-like greens."

"--and from vitamin pills," says Lear.

Henry nods but goes on. "The book cautions that excessive intakes of some vitamins create toxic conditions, and that the use of supplements is about the only way one might get an excess."

"Or get enough," says Lear.

"Here is something else that I find intriguing. I mentioned carrots and leafy vegetables as sources of vitamin A, but that's not all. 'Biologically active carotenoids are found in carrots and dark green leafy vegetables . . . [and] most carotenoids,...trap free radicals. . . .'"

"Stop right there! I've been thinking about free radicals," says Victor. "I'm beginning to sense that combating free radicals may be one of the most important things we can do to slow the aging process."

"You're right," says Henry. "I've already told you I regularly take antioxidants--C, E, beta carotene in vitamin A, and selenium. May not need them, may take more than needed, but if I could take only one thing, it would be antioxidants. I think free radicals are our slow killers.

"Now, let's look at vitamin D, like A, fat-soluble. You get vitamin D from the sun or a tanning lamp, but that depends on how much skin is exposed, and our other advice is to avoid the sun. No one of us has ever taken that advice, so I reckon we get enough vitamin D.

"The other source is various vegetables, which got it from the ultraviolet rays of the sun, and eggs that get it from I know not where.

"Rickets and other bone disorders come from a vitamin D deficiency. That is rare, now. Milk, you'll note on the carton, is usually fortified with vitamin D, as are other foods."

"Fortified makes milk the same as a vitamin pill," says Lear.

"Now, let me mention vitamin E. For our purposes this is a tocopherol--the chemistry name--that is the type most found in nature--meaning vegetable oils, wheat germ, nuts, green leafy vegetables. Meat, fish, fruits, vegetables have a little.

"The tocopherols, including vitamin E, are antioxidants, which we believe are good medicine for free radicals, Vic, and, to quote from the book, 'Vitamin E is the primary defense against potentially harmful oxidations.' It also serves other needs. Adults tolerate oral doses of vitamin E of 800 IU a day, but the book says there is a lack of evidence of a need for supplements, and recommends 10 IU per day."

"Lack of evidence!" howls Lear. "You need vitamin E, so why not take a little pill each day to be sure?"

"I haven't disagreed," says Henry.

Will Mack says, "Thank you, Henry. I have a feeling that vitamin E has an important role in slowing aging."

"The RDA people haven't learned that," says Lear.

"Let's keep our focus. We are talking about the several vitamins. Now for vitamin K," Henry proceeds. "It is also fat soluble, and according to the book, a deficiency relates in a major way only to coagulation of the blood. It has some other minor functions, apparently.

"It is manufactured in some vague degree by intestinal bacteria, but that is not enough, and small amounts come from milk, meats, eggs, cereals, fruits, and vegetables.

"You all realize this is a fairly technical book, and I am trying to pick out only what I think we need to know."

"Sounds good," says Zaroom. "Move it on, Doc."

"Okay, here is vitamin C, the glamour gal of vitamins. It was first discovered as the missing part of the diet that caused people, mostly sailors, to have scurvy, a disease of collagen, thus a fourth cousin of arthritis."

"Henry," asks, Will Mack, "do you know why British sailors are called 'Limeys'?"

"Well, no. But we need a break from this alphabet lesson."

"Oh no. It's a relevant point. In the last part of the last century, when the cause of scurvy was first suspected, sailors in the Royal Navy were issued limes to supply what was later identified as vitamin C. They first were called lime-juicers."

"They were also issued a jigger of grog," adds Lear.

"Great way to keep body and soul together. No wonder they ruled the seas."

"Anyhow, they call them limeys, not groggies."

"Very well," Henry continues, "and vitamin C has been assigned new duties over the years. You remember that Norman Cousins gave vitamin C credit for saving his life. The big book cites as additional values of vitamin C, the body's defense systems, wound healing, immune responses, formation of collagen, and as involved with many other substances in various enzyme actions."

"All that," says Lear, "and the RDA people recommend just enough to stop scurvy?"

"Does seem that they missed the boat. The body cannot manufacture vitamin C, as important as it is. It comes from foods, from citrus fruits, potatoes, and other vegetables, and smaller amounts from meats, eggs, milk, poultry, and fish. There is no vitamin C in grains."

"And I would bet a fair amount comes from vitamin tablets," says Lear.

"No doubt, and the book says vitamin C supplements are taken by 35 percent of adults in the United States. It does take another pass at the subject by noting that only about 3000 mg can be stored if the daily intake is 200 mg or more. The implication is that additional doses are simply passed through the bladder.

"The book asserts, rather defensively it seems, that 'The dietary allowances for vitamin C must be set, rather arbitrarily, between the amount necessary to prevent . . . scurvy (10 mg per day) and the amount beyond which the bulk of vitamin C is . . . excreted . . . (approximately 200 mg per day).'"

"The book, after much explanation, recommends the RDA for vitamin C at 60 mg per day, which would store enough so that, if stopped, 'this level of intake will prevent the signs of scurvy for at least 4 weeks.' And they add, 'an intake of 60 mg is easily provided in ordinary mixed diets.'"

"Only 60--why not 200?"

"There is a constant bias against vitamin tablets, isn't there?" says Rodney.

"Well, you're getting it Roddy," says Lear. "I want more than a four-week scurvy cushion. Besides, vitamin C has lots more to do than prevent scurvy? Those people are behind the times."

"Yes," says Joe Zaroom. "What about big doses of vitamin C for colds. I like that."

"You hit the raw nerve. The book mentions Linus Pauling, who is the champion of that. They say all this is not proven, and 'Routine use of larger doses of ascorbic acid is therefore not recommended.'"

"As you know, Henry," says Will Mack, "I've been reading Pauling's book. I'll let you know his arguments. I'll tell you this: He is a feisty gent."

"Okay, I need to hurry on," says Henry. "But first, let me mention a less official book. I also have studied *Food and Nutrition*. This book is very good, by the editors of *Prevention*, a magazine published by Rodale Press. It covers a discussion of nutrients, of fiber, fat, antioxidants, harmful food additives, among numerous other things we've talked about.

"They give us 'Five Steps to An Anti-Aging Diet' which I believe is sound. I will sum up the first four: Decrease fat to less than 30 percent of daily calories, increase fiber, eat foods rich in antioxidants, and consume low fat foods high in calcium.

"That fits the eat right part of our Final Four," says Joe.

"Then, for number five, get this: 'Take a multivitamin/mineral supplement to ensure you're getting at least the Recommended Dietary Allowance.'"

"There you are!" explains Lear.

"Sure, okay," Henry goes on, "Let me mention quickly there are needs for thiamin, riboflavin, and niacin, vitamins of the B complex, but I'll just leave it at that unless someone wants me to read from the Big Book about them."

"Roll on, O mighty Mississippi!" says Joe.

"Okay, we come to vitamin B-6. Important. Essential for the proper metabolism of the amino acids, so the more proteins you eat, the more B-6 you need. But vitamin B-6 is contained in the proteins that need B-6 for metabolism of their amino acids."

"So. Meat is fortified by nature with B-6?"

"The trouble is that vitamin B-6 is a fickle mate. It easily escapes in processing. So it might not be there for the meat it is supposed to accompany."

"What happens if amino acids don't get metabolized?" asks Will Mack. "Is an adequate amount of vitamin B-6 essential?"

"If we cook it out, how do we get it back?" asks Lear.

"You tell us, professor," says Zaroom.

"One obvious way is to take a supplement," says Will. "What happens if we don't?"

"The point is," Henry picks up, "that if amino acids are not metabolized, what happens? What are the negative results of a deficiency of vitamin B-6? I long ago read of a British study that B-6 was the most important nutrient for keeping cholesterol from clogging your valves, which they related to amino acids causing vascular damage. I believe vitamin B-6 plays a role in protecting the cardiovascular system, that partially converted amino acids harm the blood vessels. There is little I could find in the U.S. literature but the British theory relates the cause of vascular damage to un-processed amino acids. This calls forth a coating of the damaged area by cholesterol as a relief process, which in turn catches addi-tional cholesterol that blocks blood flow and brings about heart at-tacks. My RDA book on page 337 notes that dietary vitamin B-6 is rapidly converted by the liver into an coenzyme, which has a con-trol role in the metabolism of amino acids. I've been taking a B-6 supplement for a dozen years and I've got a fairly high cholesterol count but my veins are absolutely clean. I realize that doesn't prove anything to science, but it does to me.'"

"Wow," says Joe. "Sounds like a spy novel."

"Anyhow, it is my considered conclusion," Henry continues, "that the B-6 is one of the major vitamins we need, and, you'll be pleased to know, Lear, that we can't be sure that we get enough in the ordinary American diet. We need a B-6 supplement."

"Foolish not to buy that insurance."

"Another theory, let me quote from page 337, 'a vitamin B-6 de-ficiency, at a critical time during cell division could result in indi-vidual mutations that develop into a tumor.' The author suggests that dietary vitamin B-6 supplementation could assist in preventing some cancers.'"

"Good. They are making progress."

"Also, 'Vitamin B-6 is involved in the synthesis of DNA bases.' On page 330: 'Vitamin B-6 dependent enzymes are needed...most of which involve amino acid metabolism.' On page 441: 'Vitamin B-6 plays an important role in the production of antibody response to various antigens.'"

"The conclusion is that B-6 may be as special as vitamins C and E."

"Now let me jump back to *Prevention*'s book, *Food and Nutrition*. They tell us that 'the needs of younger adults are not the same as those of people in their sixties, seventies, and eighties. Take the vi-tamin B-6 study as an example. While it was only a preliminary study, it does suggest the need for vitamin B-6 may increase with age . . .might prevent or delay age-related changes in the immune system."

"I like all that," says Will. "I'm glad I take B-6."

"Fair enough. Next is vitamin B-12. It comes primarily from synthesization by bacteria, fungi, and algae, and gets into the body through animal products where it has accumulated."

"Ugh," says Joe.

"A shortage results in anemia, but shortages are rare. Does it have positive functions? I think so."

"I think the whole B-complex is important," says Will Mack. Too important to leave to chance."

"I agree and I have a few more. Folate, similar to folic acid, a B-complex vitamin. This is found in leafy vegetables, peanuts, beans and grains, but the National Academy of Sciences book tells us that heat destruction in cooking causes high losses. A deficiency leads to impaired cell division. We need to worry about cell division at our age."

"Meaning, get Folate in your daily vitamin tablet," says Lear.

"That's my view. Of the needed minerals, the principal one is calcium, which is needed by the bones, especially for women, and the calcium in fluids and cell membranes has an essential role in muscle contraction and other functions. We need an adequate amount for bone health, and maybe other things."

"Yes," says Victor, "I read in the newspaper that an NIH study indicates that we have put too much emphasis on cutting down on salt to guard against hypertension, when it turns out that the danger is not too much salt, but too little calcium."

"Sure, and Fries and Vickery suggest we need 1000 mg of calcium a day, so maybe we need a few calcium antacid tablets every day, or other source of a calcium supplement."

"Of course we do," says Lear.

"It is generally recommended that women take calcium supplements as they get older," says Victor, "but I don't know what your RDA book says about it."

"Not much. But you are right, adequate calcium is a guard against osteoporosis, and the *Prevention* book recommends calcium supplements especially for women.

"The other minerals recognized by RDA standards are phosphorus and magnesium, both of which are essential to a number of body processes.

"Then there are the trace elements, iron, zinc, iodine, selenium, copper, manganese, fluoride, chromium, and molybdenum."

"Sounds like a space ship," says Joe.

"Not enough of all of them to weigh you down, but the little traces have countless life-promoting qualities. You'll find them in most combined vitamin tablets.

"That's it, fellows, for the RDA book. I have another big book, covering much of the same, and we could spend a month studying it."

"Why don't we," asks Joe.

"It is too technical, too lengthy, and I didn't promise to make nutritionists and dietitians out of you. This is a remarkably thorough report by the National Research Council, actually it's Committee on Health and Diet, titled *Diet and Health*, with 'Implications for Reducing Chronic Disease Risk,' and the National Research Council, organized in 1916, is made up of members drawn from the National Academy of Science, the National Academy of Engineering, and the Institute of Medicine."

"Wow!" gasps Joe.

"Some credentials," says Will Mack.

"The book confirms much of what we have learned. When related to a number of chronic diseases, saturated fats are potentially harmful, fruits, vegetables, cereals, and legumes are generally beneficial, and a high protein diet can increase risks."

"We know that about saturated fats."

"Sure. I have gone to this authoritative report to pick up its views on vitamins and supplements.

"First, and I quote, 'The potential risks or benefits of the long term use of small doses of supplements have not been systematically examined.'"

"Why not?"

"They're getting to it, and this Report recommends much specific research.

"We can't wait."

"Now, they report, 'The special dietary needs of the elderly are largely unknown."

"So we have to figure it out for ourselves?"

"Yes, but with some encouragement. Hear this, from page 513: 'Several studies show, however, that the diets of many elderly people fail to meet the RDAs for several nutrients--including calcium, zinc, vitamins B-6, and iron and...many elderly people are at risk of nutrient deficiencies for reasons that include physiological decline, poor economic status, inadequate food intake, disease processes, and medical treatments.'"

"Well, there you are!" Lear slaps the table.

"Why take chances on being at risk?" asks Victor.

"Now, they point out that healthy adults should obtain adequate vitamins from diet, but, they edge up on the subject most cautiously, 'Supplement usage may be indicated in some circumstances.'"

"May be indicated...good progress!"

"They're getting there," says Lear.

"Not quite. They are quoting a recommendation by the American Dietetic Association, American Society for Clinical Nutrition, American Institute of Nutrition and the National Council Against Health Fraud. Their 'circumstances' do not cover older people as such, although it is clear our special needs have not been studied adequately, if at all. They do concede supplements are justified 'for some vegetarians' and 'people with very low caloric intakes.'"

"That's a step forward," says Lear.

"Barely, but let me put into evidence the word of *Food and Nutrition*: 'But there is a growing number of studies that the RDAs are not really appropriate or sensitive to the changing nutritional needs of aging adults. Nor are they focused on our most important public health objectives--preventing chronic disease like cancer and heart disease.'"

"I like this attitude," says Lear.

"All right. Do we get these by supplements, by vitamin tablets?" asks Victor.

"It may be a debatable question, but you know I've been taking them," Henry pronounces.

"Damn right," says Lear.

"I say certain ones," says Will Mack.

"Of course," says Victor.

"Silly not to," says Joe Zaroom.

"Well," says Roddy, "I'll keep an open mind."

"I know you will," Henry nods,

"Good job," Henry, "we've learned a lot. Time to go?"

"I suppose so. See you next week. You ready with your feisty friend, Will?"

"I'll be ready."

Chapter Seventeen

LINUS PAULING--TELLS IT LIKE IT IS

*V*iolet has served the coffee when Henry arrives, the last of the group. "Violet," he says, "You looked stunning at the Eldorado Restaurant last night. I didn't know he was your beau."

"Don't you tell them who I was with," Violet stuttered.

"Is he serious?"

"He better be serious. He's slippery, but I've 'bout got him ready to pop the question. After we had dinner and danced a little, he brought me home and came in the house but Mama came in to see if everything was all right, wanted to know if he wanted some of her cookies and milk. I'm beginning to suspicion that Mama don't want me getting married."

"Bring him by my house next time and we'll lock him in until he proposes."

"Well now, ver-ry in-ter-rest-ing," says Will. "Tell us more."

"Tell you nothing. It might jinx me. Don't tell 'em, Mr. Henry. Let me have your orders."

Before Violet returns, Henry points to Will. "Mack has the class today. He read a story about Linus Pauling, saw he had written a book named *How to Live Longer and Feel Better*, and volunteered to get it from the library. Ready to go, Mack?"

"Sure. I can eat corn flakes and talk at the same time. Article was by Christine Russell in the *Washington Post*. Pauling is a remarkable man, two Nobel Prizes, one for science and one for peace.

He is known in science as a giant in chemistry, known by the public as a political activist against nuclear testing.

"So you wouldn't be surprised that the last sentence in his book is: 'Do not let either the medical authorities or the politicians mislead you. Find out what the facts are, and make your own decisions about how to live a happy life and how to work for a better world.'"

"That's my man!" exclaims Lear.

"How true, how true! I'll buy that," says Vic Beane.

"I do too," Will Mack continues. "And also apply it to car salesmen and stock brokers. But let me tell you about his views on gaining a healthy old age, which the book is about.

"He has some original and controversial views. You might not agree, and it is not up to me to sell you on what he contends, but I have a tremendous respect for his intellect. He is spry into his nineties, and the newspaper article was about that.

"His book makes his case for vitamins, that vitamins are needed in optimum amounts, especially vitamin C and he recommends a minimum of 6,000 milligrams of vitamin C every day.

"He takes 12,000 milligrams of ascorbic acid, vitamin C, every morning."

"That is mighty high," says Lear. "Even I can see how other scientists would scream."

"So high I started not to tell you.

"He says he cannot prove his estimate, but contends that the optimum amount of vitamin C and other vitamins he writes about will increase the immune system and the natural protective mechanisms of the body. As you might guess, many scientists do not accept Pauling's theory of vitamin C.

"I'll buy the theory, not the amount. I believe we know that about nine-tenths of that much will surely wash out," says Victor.

"No argument," Will Mack responds." I think the lesson is to get an ample amount which is probably nothing like the amount Pauling takes. But he is making his point about the value of vitamin C."

"It's a good point."

"Now do you think meats and fats get a bum rap for causing heart attacks, Rodney?"

"I didn't--until you mentioned it. Are you kidding?"

"Linus Pauling believes it."

"Okay. What's his proof?"

"It ain't simple. Let me try. I've made notes.

"First of all he debunks the cholesterol theories. Eat eggs and meat, he suggests. He affirms that diet and heart disease are related, along with our affluent and sedentary lifestyles. But listen to this: 'cholesterol is a lipid, soluble in fats and oils . . . manufactured in all cells of animals, especially the liver. . . . Human beings synthesize about 3000 to 4000 milligrams per day and receive a somewhat smaller amount in their food, mainly from eggs and meat. Cholesterol is found in all the tissues of the human body, especially the brain and the spinal cord. . . . [and] people with a high percentage of cholesterol in the blood have an increased incidence of cardiovascular disease."

"I've listened carefully. So far that seems to be what I've heard from my doctor," says Rodney. "Except for eating the eggs and meat."

"Okay, now for his next point. 'It has now been found that the incidence of cardiovascular disease tends to increase with increase in the amounts of total blood cholesterol, low-density lipoprotein (LDL) cholesterol, and triglycerides (little fatty particles), and--understand this--high-density lipoprotein (HDL) cholesterol will decrease the likelihood of the disease.'"

"I know all that," says Rodney. "Why should we not cut down eating eggs and meat, which contain cholesterol?"

"Ah, there's his departure," says Will Mack. "Recapitulate. The amount of cholesterol in the bloodstream is determined by four things: How much is synthesized in the liver, how much comes from food, how much of this is converted into bile acids, and the amount of bile acids reabsorbed through the bowels and reconverted into cholesterol. Stay with me, Roddy, I'm getting there."

"Doesn't that prove we should cut down on eating cholesterol and saturated fats?" Rodney insists.

"Now, hear this from Pauling: 'But it has been known since 1970 from the multi-million-dollar Framingham study of diet and heart disease that restricting the intake of cholesterol does not reduce the cholesterol level in the blood.'"

"Wait a dadgummed minute," says Rodney. "How, then, do we reduce this danger? What does his eminence offer?"

"He says much more cholesterol comes from the liver than from food, and that 'the fat-in-food-cholesterol-the-bloodstream idea is dying hard. . . . During the last decade it has become increasingly evident that the great hope of thirty years ago that heart disease could be controlled by limiting the intake of saturated fat (as in meat and butter) and cholesterol (in meat and eggs) and increasing that of unsaturated fat . . . (margarine, certain vegetable oils) had failed.'"

"Ah, so. Failed? Plow on," says Rodney

"So the liver manufactures the excess? Is that what he's saying?" Vic asks.

"He was working his way toward this shocker. Hear this--' . . . it is the increase in consumption of sugar sucrose that has brought on the pandemic of heart and circulatory disease in the prosperous industrial countries of the world.'"

"Sugar!" exclaims Joe.

"Well, I'll be damned. It is pecan pie and ice cream, not sausage and eggs." Rodney gave a long mock sigh.

"I can't handle it," says Lear.

"Remember, Henry mentioned sugar as a possible suspect."

"He sure did. Now I'm telling you what Pauling said. The liver manufactures cholesterol from acetate--which is provided by fructose and other precursors. Here we go.

"Ordinary sugar when ingested forms equal amounts of glucose and fructose.

"Glucose is what forms from the vegetable and fruit starches we eat, and these small molecules pass through the walls of the intestines and are transmitted to cells by the bloodstream and are burned to provide energy.

"Fructose also comes in relatively small amounts from fruits and honey, about 8 grams a day, according to Dr. Pauling not enough to cause any trouble. Then with the advent of sugar cane and sugar beets, Dr. Pauling reports, the daily intake of fructose rose tenfold, to about 75 grams per day. Today, he says, the American diet gets 20 percent of the food energy from sucrose--sugars, that is.

"Does he include all the corn sweeteners in everything, especially in soda pop," asks Lear.

"I'd guess so. He says we are taking in far higher amounts of fructose, and fructose is a precursor of cholesterol. I quote: 'Fructose metabolism goes in part by a different route such that it produces acetate, which is a precursor of the cholesterol that we synthesize in our liver cells.'

"What are the other precursors? Fat?"

"Probably, but he doesn't say. Maybe Henry can find out."

"He writes that 'It has been shown in a trustworthy clinical study that the ingestion of sucrose leads to an increase in the cholesterol concentration in the blood.'

"Let me tell you about that experiment. Eighteen male subjects were 'in a locked ward,'--in prison, I presume--and were fed a rigidly controlled diet. The first four weeks was described as 'ordinary food.' Then, for four weeks the carbohydrate ingredient was glucose along with protein and essential fats. No sugar. The cholesterol levels in all eighteen fell from an average of 227 (mg. per deciliter) to 173 in two weeks, and to 160 in another two weeks.

"Then for four weeks the carbohydrate part of the diet was changed to 75 percent glucose and 25 percent sucrose (sugar). The cholesterol average jumped back up to 208.

"For the fourth stage the glucose, no-sugar diet was resumed, and over six weeks the cholesterol average leveled at 150."

"Pretty good evidence, I'd say," says Lear.

"Maybe. Certainly should have prompted some follow-up," notes Victor.

"Pauling cites one other piece of evidence--a study some twenty years ago by a London professor, John Yudkin--published in a book entitled *Sweet and Dangerous*.

"Yudkin contended that the correlation between the intake of sugar and coronary disease is much better than the correlation with fat consumption. He stated that 'no one has ever shown any difference in fat consumption between people with and people without coronary diseases. . . .'"

"As I remember, Henry, the Farmingham man blamed this on the excess sugars being burned more quickly than fats, leaving fats to be stored and to clog the veins."

"That's right. Different reasons, they both blame sugar."

"Well, we need to look for more information. What does your big RDA and Health and Diet Books say about sugar, Henry?" asks Victor.

"Not much," says Henry. "Causes tooth decay, they warn. Doesn't get into the path sugars take in the body. The *Prevention* book says, empty calories, "and suggests, 'protect your waistline, get your sugars the natural way--from grapes, watermelon and other fruits.'

Then Rodney asks, "But the evidence is pretty slim, and the claim has been around twenty years or more, and the official advice from the government and doctors is still to cut down on cholesterol foods and fats. Pauling cites only a couple of studies. I never before heard of sugar as the culprit. How come?'"

"Pauling would say that the medical establishment is bull-headed," says Will Mack.

"And the sugar lobby? Do the Department of Agriculture nutritionists have an official view?"

"Some might say that the Agriculture Department has too much at stake with the sugar and corn growers. They don't want to know about sugars increasing cholesterol."

"That's cynical, Lear," says Roddy.

"Sure is," retorts Lear.

"I can tell you others do not agree with Linus," says Henry. "Danger of sugar? At worst, causes tooth decay they say. I can't find any official source that deals with sugar and cholesterol."

"But let me read how he drove home his sugar belief: ' . . . as to eating and drinking there is in this book only one real *don't*; that is sugar. Like the cigarette, the sugar sucrose is a novelty of industrial civilization. Together, they have brought pandemics of cancer and cardiovascular disease to the otherwise fortunate populations of the developed countries. . . . Sucrose cannot be avoided, but a larger decrease in the intake of sugar is essential.'"

"He sure ain't tentative," says Lear.

"He's tough," says Rodney.

"All right, now listen to another value he attributes to vitamin C. Here it is: 'If you keep your intake of sugar down, vitamin C can supply the rest of your insurance against high cholesterol concentration in your bloodstream.'"

"Proof?" asks Rodney.

"Maybe. HDL cholesterol, you remember, is the good kind, a preventative for cardiovascular disease. Dr. Pauling reports studies that 'an increased intake of vitamin C increases the HDL level.'"

"Good. But you said it would decrease cholesterol."

"Indeed. He reports 'that vitamin C has little effect on the cholesterol level in the normal range, below about 200 mg per deciliter, but has a large effect in decreasing high levels by 10 to 20 percent.'"

"Ten to twenty. Not bad."

"But not good enough by itself. Let me sum up what he says, from page 149: 'Along with the reduction of sucrose in the diet there is another measure everyone can take to reduce the risk of heart disease from elevated cholesterol levels in the blood: . . . . an increase intake of vitamin C decreases total cholesterol, LDL cholesterol, and triglycerides, and increases HDL cholesterol. . . .' One way C works is to increase the conversion of cholesterol into bile acids."

"Okay, Will, good job. Is there anything else?"

"He writes that 'persons with a tendency toward arthritis might benefit by increases in vitamin C, niacinamide, and vitamin B-6.' And I am leaving out a sizable part of his book."

"I believe he is right about arthritis," says Victor.

"All right," says Rodney, "but all this is not for certain, not fully proven, is it?"

"You can say that. But he has thrown down some red meat for the scientists."

"Something else," says Lear, "is that I can do without sweets. But you can't get away from it. Sugar is in just about everything on the grocery shelves. Even vegetable soup and biscuit mix. I'll bet we will find that this sugar business has been one massive cover up. We got too much financial interest to mess with sugar."

"You admit you are a bit of a cynic, Lear?" asks Will Mack, smiling.

"Of course I am!"

"Pauling's main theme is, ' . . . thanks to the new science of nutrition, you can today multiply the benefits of healthy habits by taking, every day, the optimum amounts of the essential vitamins.'"

"So, what is optimum?"

"I'll not go through all his numbers, but he takes vitamin C, E, D, A, super-B, folacin, pantothentic acid, B-12/B-3, and a multi-mineral tablet. He takes four tablets plus ascorbic acid crystals, some in the morning, some at night. Says you can get them from a good pharmaceutical company--it costs him 41 cents a day.

"He's not into ginsing, garlic, and bee pollen, I might note, and he cautions not to go beyond the RDA for minerals which might be toxic in large amounts."

"Anything else in Pauling's regimen?"

"Oh, yes. Vitamins are his game, but he mentions several other things, including to avoid stress, to like your job, and 'be happy with your family.'

"Fair enough. What else?"

"He again hits sugar. We average one hundred pounds a year, he says. Cut it in half. Much of it is converted to cholesterol, and manufacturers seem to put it into everything.

"I'm quitting now. I'm out of breath."

"Well done!" Henry claps.

"Remarkable. Fresh thinking. Makes sense," says Victor.

"You said he was feisty," says Roddy.

"Time to go, I reckon," says Henry. "See you next week.

"I've got to go by the store and get some diet drinks," says Roddy.

Chapter Eighteen

VITAMINS FOR OLDER PEOPLE-- CAUTIONS

*V*iolet had taken the orders and was now clearing the dishes.

"Will," says Rodney, "I said that I didn't want to accept all Dr. Pauling says about vitamins. He is a scientist. Did he prove all he claims?"

"No. And he didn't claim he had, as I read him," retorts Will Mack.

Henry takes charge. "I've come loaded for your questions about vitamins. So we can measure this against Dr. Pauling's views. Let me refer to some notes.

"Let me start with the Surgeon General's 1988 Report on Nutrition and Health. Right from the book, specifically on the subject of aging people: 'Whether such supplements improve the health of these people cannot be determined from existing data, . . . '"

"That seems unbelievable," says Victor. "In all the research, why hasn't all of our government looked at the needs of older people?"

"They are just beginning to notice that people get older."

"Fair enough. Let me read from the same book which tells us that a study 'indicated that the persons most likely to take supplemental nutrients are less likely to need them, and those most in need of them are least likely to take them. . . .'"

"There they go again," says Lear. "An admission that people need vitamins. Why don't they just quit hedging?"

"Well, maybe they do, Lear. They note that the older 'population requires special consideration because aging per se changes the absorption, disposition, and elimination of drugs.'

"And they go on to say that the older persons who cannot or do not get adequate nutrients in their food 'should receive advice on the proper type and dosage of nutrient supplements. Such supplements may be appropriate for some older persons. . . .'"

"Right! Finally that is official advice," says Will Mack.

"Not so fast," drawls Lear. "Where are they going to get good advice? The doctors don't know much about vitamins. Why can't the Surgeon General just give clear, honest advice?"

"Maybe they're learning that older people have different vitamin needs," says Rodney. "You know I've been talking to my doctor, telling him I've been defending him, and he pretty nearly admitted last Saturday that he had not been giving me the most thoughtful advice. Said the medical fraternity had been irritated by the fraud in advertising of all kinds of supplements, reducing potions, and so on, and had let their bias keep them from confronting the issue.

"And I told him that I thought older people got taken in by the hucksters because they sense that they need to round out their nutrients, and the medical profession isn't giving what appears to be a sensible response."

"You're right," says Victor. "Older people don't believe you are likely to get a balanced diet including all the recommended daily allowances. Makes sense. We know there's no such thing as a uniformly balanced diet. Most people don't know what one is and couldn't be sure even if they were experts. So they figure it out on their own, and their best source of information is the paid advertisements by the hucksters. No wonder they buy all kinds of needless pills and powders."

"And," adds Will Mack, "the recommended daily allowance, the famous RDA, was not set for the needs of older people."

"Right on the target," says Henry. "Let me tell you about Nancy Chapman, a registered dietitian. In a paper for the National Institute on Aging, she reports that older people are eager to control their health, are confused about the contradictory claims about nutrition, and, in her words, 'find physicians generally not knowledgeable about nutrition and somewhat impersonal, and therefore don't rely on physicians for dietary advice.'"

"That's my point," says Rodney, "and I have the utmost respect for my doctor. If the National Institute on Aging would endorse appropriate supplement use, and if doctors were more open on the question, we might not all have to be confused by all the self-serving advertisements."

"I agree," says Henry, "but even if they were open-minded, there is a lot not known. I've got a note here from the *Diet and Health* book of the National Academy of Sciences which points up the problem. This is just one example. Two points. 'Although there are ample data on nutrients in commodities, there is little information on highly processed or manufactured foods such as snack foods, baked products, convenience foods, restaurant meals, and frozen dinners. . . .'"

"You have just covered our monthly menu," says Rodney. "If we are not microwaving it, we are thawing it or we are ordering a pizza or going to a restaurant or driving through a quick food."

"I hear you. Let me finish the quote. 'In addition, knowledge is limited regarding the amounts of vitamin B-6, pantothentic acid, folacin, vitamin E, zinc, copper, magnesium, manganese, chromium, and selenium in foods.'"

"In other words, they have the obvious in various foods, A, B, C, and so on, but not all the necessary nutrients. Where do you get the necessary B-6 and selenium, and minerals, how much do you need, why do you need them?

"And we can," says Will Mack, "if we want to, wait around until they study all there is to know about diets, and then we won't be here to hear about it. We just need a clear, non-evasive, un-hedged policy about how to take vitamin supplements for preventive health care as we grow older. It seems so simple."

"And I ain't got time to wait."

"You are right about that, Lear. Let me read on. Chapman says, 'Compared to non-users, supplement users have a better profile of health promoting behaviors overall.'"

"Of course they do. They are the ones who are making the conscious effort to stay in good health."

"Sure, and she says, 'Supplement users smoke less, weigh less, exercise more, and eat more nutritious diets.'"

"But Henry, you--she--doesn't suggest that the vitamins don't matter, that the reason for better health is the other behavior?"

"Oh no, not at all. Her subject is vitamin supplements. She is saying the savvy ones, the ones paying attention to aging, take their vitamin supplements."

"Like I told my dear friend, Dr. Gibson, the doctors need to be more candid, less afraid of breaking from convention, more concerned about the fears and hopes of older people who want to stay in the best health possible." Rodney shakes his head in puzzlement.

"What did Gibby say to that?"

"He didn't disagree."

"Okay, but before you get carried away, most doctors, all I suppose, insist that you need the RDA, the recommended daily allowances."

"Sure they do. Two things wrong with that advice," says Joe. "You need a little more than RDA as you grow older--absorption and so on. Second, you can't for sure eat a balanced diet."

"You're right about that," says Henry. "I can quote from Nancy's report that the RDA 'allowances may not adequately reflect the specific needs of the elderly population, and need to be examined more closely.'"

"And the RDA figures are low," says Lear. "They've got vitamin C set just high enough to keep you from getting scurvy when there is plenty of evidence that vitamin C has antioxidant qualities, and many other needed purposes."

"Maybe helps with arthritis."

"Okay, okay. Let me quote her again. 'Older people must meet the same (or perhaps higher) nutrient levels than younger adults but with fewer calories. They often fall short of meeting the RDAs through dietary intakes alone. Ryan and Bower estimate that inadequate nutrient intake accounts for one-third to one-half of the health problems of the elderly.'"

"Read it again!"

"Gosh," says Joe, "that's strong stuff."

"That's convincing," says Roddy.

"Sure is," Henry continues. "A couple of more words from Nancy Chapman. An increase over the RDA for vitamin A may provide disease protection, and adequate vitamin E 'may improve immune function and help elderly resist disease.' I'd say there is not any question that older people ought to have their own regimen of vitamin supplements."

"But Henry, at the established RDAs?"

"No! She says avoid megadoses, but it is clear to me that RDA's are inadequate for older people. Official word!"

"So," says Will Mack. "I'm not taking a chance. I'll continue to take a daily supplement, with a little augmentation where I see fit, and I hope that the powers-that-be will come up with some sound advice for people who are getting older. Why wait for my children to note in later years of what might have been? I expect to be here when I am 110 bragging on what I learned from Henry Murphy's readings."

"Well, I can't take issue with your testimonial," says Henry, "The scientific community has sort of left us older citizens to make our own decisions, I'd have to admit.

"Well, let's make 'em!"

"Let me add one last thing that is important. Even if we are not satisfied with the physicians and the scientific community on the matter of nutrients, be wary of large doses. Nancy Chapman says that and it also comes from the Surgeon General's Report. And it is good sense."

"I can buy that," says Will.

"And Nancy Chapman has a few more cautions, and lists some no-noes. Don't spend money for aloe vera, bee pollen, brewer's yeast in excess, fiber in excess, flavonoids, garlic oil, ginsing, herbal preparations, inositol, and laetrile; and avoid nightshades, poke root, spiruline, raw glandular concentrates, snake venom, all of which might or might not be harmful, but certainly are not useful."

"All right, all of that is good," says Roddy, "and it is maybe useless for me to talk about this paper that Charlie sent me. The *Age Page* on supplements. They beat around the bush. They are too concerned with megadoses and excesses that they fail to give the advice the ordinary elderly person needs."

"You're about to become an evangelist, Roddy."

"Maybe. They do say that many people take these vitamin pills and minerals as a form of 'insurance' that their daily nutritional needs are met. I'm an insurance man."

"Of course they take it as insurance," says Lear. "Why doesn't the establishment admit this is good? Beating around the bush!"

"The *Age Page* goes on, 'A well-balanced diet--one that contains a wide variety of foods--provides all the necessary nutrients,' including..."

"That is doubtless true, but it begs the question," Will Mack interrupts. "What is this diet? How do we get it? Can most people keep to it? Do older people have special needs?'"

"Well, they tell us, ' . . . at least two servings of milk or dairy products such as cheese, cottage cheese, or yogurt. . . .'"

"Wait a minute there. We have been told to avoid the fats in cheeses."

"'Two servings of lean meat. . . .'"

"Wait a minute. They want us to limit our meats to 4 ounces a day."

"' . . .poultry, fish, eggs. . . .'"

"Wait a minute, eggs are limited because of cholesterol."

"'Beans, nuts, or peanut butter; four servings of fruits and vegetables, including a citrus fruit or juice and a dark-green leafy vegetable; and four servings of breads and cereal products made with whole grain or enriched flours. . . .'"

"Wait a minute--enriched with what--vitamin supplements?"

"' . . . rice, or pasta.' Whew!"

"You want to run through that again?" asks Lear.

"Heavens no. I've never done such broken field running just to read one sentence. Will is a great defensive player."

"Well," says Will Mack, "I can't stand double talk.

"Now Henry, you know I have a series of papers presented by the New York Academy of Science on the use of vitamins. This is the best research I have seen, and I want to give us a summary of what they report."

"Sure," says Henry, "Tell where you got them."

"Ethel read a press release that scientists at an international conference said that better vitamin nutrition would soon be recognized as an important part of the prevention and treatment of disease, so she ordered copies. The New York Academy of Science, I found out, is 175 years old and a highly regarded international organization. I believe this is the latest word on vitamins.

"Let me read from my highlights. I've got all the summaries of their papers for anyone who wants to see them.

"Dr. DeLuca, distinguished research professor and chairman of Biochemistry at the University of Wisconsin-Madison, who we are told is 'the preeminent authority on vitamin D metabolism,' reports that 'New research has shown that vitamin D, whose major roles include maintaining calcium levels in the blood stream, building bones and preventing rickets, may play a role in suppressing the growth of cancer cells.' He pointedly does not suggest excessive doses.

"Dr. Gladys Block, professor at the School of Public Health at the University of California, Berkeley, has reported that 'Epidimiologic and biochemical data indicate that vitamin C plays an important role in cancer prevention.'

"Let me read more fully from the abstract of her paper: 'Ascorbic acid (vitamin C) acts as an antioxidant in the blood stream, neutralizing oxygen-containing particles called free radicals that are formed in the body and can damage cells. Cell damage is thought to be one of the first steps in the development of cancer. Vitamin C also works together with vitamin E, another antioxidant vitamin found in cells, to help restore vitamin E's ability to function as an antioxidant.'"

"That confirms what Henry has already told us."

"Exactly!" Will Mack continues. "I have the abstracts from a dozen papers delivered at this conference--by very distinguished scientists. Some are not prepared to make final conclusions, but they are on the trail of something important.

"Here is C.E. Butterworth, M.D., of the Department of Nutrition Sciences at the University of Alabama at Birmingham, whose paper 'implies that long-term improvement in nutritional intake of folic acid, and probably of other nutrients, may be protective against cervical cancer.'

"This conclusion was confirmed by Dr. Douglas Heimburger of the University of Alabama at Birmingham, who reported that folic acid supplements were beneficial in avoiding colon cancer."

"What is folic acid?" asks Joe.

"Remember," says Henry, "it is one of the nutrients, Folate, on the RDA list, one of the B vitamins. It comes from leafy vegetables and fruits and legumes, but is easily lost in cooking. Almost all daily supplements will contain at least the RDA amount."

"Okay," Will Mack goes on, "Now for another comment on cancer--this one from Dr. H.S. Garewal of the University of Arizona Cancer Center. He concludes, 'We hope and anticipate that a preventive role for beta carotene and other antioxidant nutrients against cancers of the oral cavity will emerge.'

"Now for one more. Dr. Frank L. Meyskens, Director of the Clinical Cancer Center at the University of California at Irvine, reported that 'women whose diets contained the highest amounts of beta carotene, vitamin C and/or folic acid had a lower risk of developing cervical or endometrial cancer.' Their studies of this are continuing.

"So," says Victor, "they relate our antioxidants to cancer control."

"Sure they do. Now let me tell you about heart problems and vitamins.

"Dr. Ishwarlal Jialal of the University of Texas Southwestern Medical Center reports that free radicals probably oxidize cholesterol which in turn may cause atherosclerosis. He says, 'Antioxidant nutrients, such as vitamin C, vitamin E, and beta carotene, may be instrumental in preventing LDL oxidation and subsequent atherosclerosis.' And he adds, 'levels in the body of these nutrients can be increased through diet and supplements, without the risk of side effects seen with medications.'"

"We'd be fools not to take these vitamin supplements," says Lear.

"You can believe I agree with you. Here is what Dr. Jialal says: 'Vitamin C and beta carotene almost completely inhibited LDL oxidation, (95% and 90%, respectively); vitamin E inhibited oxidation by 45%.' And, he compared vitamin C with the leading drug and found both equally effective, but 'only vitamin C preserved vitamin E and beta carotene,' and without the side effects of the drug."

"We're crazy not to take these supplements," declares Victor.

"Is all this proven?" asks Rodney, "but are these things proven?".

"Of course not," says Lear. "We send people to the gas chamber without absolute proof, but here the jury can't deny that the evidence is strong."

"I'm not disagreeing," says Roddy..

"Let me go on," says Will Mack. "Dr. Charles H. Hennekens of the Department of Preventive Medicine at Harvard Medical School reported that 'It is possible that the antioxidants beta carotene (a precursor of vitamin A that is found in many fruits and vegetables), and vitamin E may be effective in preventing or slowing the progression of atherosclerosis (hardening of the arteries).'

"In a U.S. Physicians' Health Study of 333 participants who had stable angina (chest pain) and who had not had a previous heart attack or stroke, the physicians who took 50 milligrams of beta carotene every other day had almost half as many heart attacks, strokes, and deaths related to heart disease as those who did not."

"I may have to apologize for what I have been saying about doctors," says Lear.

"And I have something else to tell my doctor," says Rodney.

"You do, indeed. Dr. Hennekens asserts that the 'preliminary data suggest that increased dietary and/or supplemental intake of certain antioxidants may be associated with reduced risk of heart disease.' He notes that more clinical trials are needed.

"And Dr. Paul F. Jacques of the Tufts University Nutrition Research Center on Aging reports that high intake of vitamin C--three times the RDA--has a 'positive effect on heart disease risk factors.'

"That's 180 mg; not high compared to Pauling's recommendations," says Rodney.

"No, but it makes the point I believe. Pauling is a little excessive, but he advocated vitamin C for more things than just heart disease. Let me conclude with one more paper.

"Dr. Simin N. Meydani, also at the Tufts University Research Center, a recognized scientist in the field of immunology, reports that the 'measures of immune response significantly improved in healthy elderly adults on 800 IU daily of vitamin E.' This is 80 times the RDA, and you will remember that vitamin C stabilizes vitamin E. She also reported the vitamin B-6 supplementation 'above the RDA' normalized 'the immune response of elderly subjects who were B-6 deficient.' That's it, Henry"

"Terrific" says Henry, "Great report, and please indulge me to go back to our concerns about senility and the wits of older people. In the *Prevention* book, Dr. Jeffrey Blumberg, associate director, USDA Human Nutrition Research Center on Aging at Tufts University, asserts '. . . to stay sharp into a ripe old age? . . . make sure that your diet is rich in. . . vitamin B-6, b-12, and Folate.'

"All these reports are remarkable, and now I think we ought to try to agree on a supplement program."

"Exciting," says Lear. "Thanks, Will."

"Convincing," says Rodney.

"Praise the Lord," says Victor. "You've convinced Roddy.

"I have some firm conclusions," says Will Mack. "Take 'em or leave 'em. One, take vitamin supplements. Second, take reasonable doses. Third, ignore all of the snake oil stuff Nancy Chapman enumerates."

"What, and how much?" asks Joe Zaroom.

"Not for me to say. I have decided to take a general component vitamin tablet, including B-complex and with minerals, every morning, plus the four antioxidants in one tablet twice a day, plus a little extra C and B-6, once a day, and maybe twice a day as I feel like it. Fairly simple. Just four bottles."

"Great finish," says Henry. "We thank you, and if there is no objection, I want to add one point.

"When I got the big report of the study by the Committee on Diet and Health, the 800-page National Science Foundation publication, I looked up sugar in the index because of Pauling. Here is what these experts say. 'Sugar consumption (by those with an adequate diet) has not been established as a risk factor for any chronic disease other than dental cavities in humans.'

"'Established,' he said?"

"Yes, but here is something else from pages 58 and 59: 'In 1909-1913, the proportion was approximately two-thirds starch and one-third sugar. By 1980, sugars furnished a little more than one-half the carbohydrates in the food supply."

"Right on! That's what Pauling said. As heart attacks increased, so did the use of sugar."

"He may be on a hot trail. Let me read. '"Because of concern about possible effects of increased fructose use on certain chronic diseases or on carbohydrate metabolism, the FDA established a Sugar Task Force to review and interpret recent relative scientific studies, and the task force pointed out the true increase in fructose availability over the past 10 years is more than the food supply data suggest, because approximately 60 percent of sucrose added to acidic beverages is converted to glucose and fructose. Such beverages consequently contain more fructose and less sucrose than food supply data indicate.'"

"Hold on," says Will Mack. "We have already learned that sucrose is converted into equal amounts of glucose and fructose in the body, so this is just saying that the acid in the beverage converts 60 percent of it ahead of time. It still ends up fructose headed for the liver."

"And cholesterol!"

"It looks that way. And here is more: '...replacement of sucrose in soft drinks and other products by corn sweeteners increased two and a half times from 1972 to 1984, and the use of high-fructose corn syrup went up 36 times, and another 20 percent a year later, meaning that sugar use has changed--from primarily sucrose to a mixture of sucrose, glucose from corn syrup, and fructose."

"Meaning more fructose for the liver?"

"That is the way I read it.

"Maybe there will be some real research on sugars."

"I hope so," says Henry. "Now, let me...

"So go with diet drinks?"

"They don't say that," Henry answers. "The connection between fructose and cholesterol has not been carefully studied."

"But it is still a big question?"

"Big question! I'd predict in their own time the experts will agree with Pauling. Sugars create cholesterol. "

"I think you are right," says Will. "Pauling instinctively comprehends many things, and there is beguiling evidence that sugars are culprits in the advance of cholesterol problems and cardiovascular disease. We'll have to wait and see."

"Meanwhile I'm drinking diet sodas," says Victor.

"Now," says Henry, "we are about to conclude this semester's work. I've got a few more rag-tags, but I've told you about all I've learned. And the rest of you have filled in a lot more. We can summarize on Monday."

"Good," says Roddy. "I've got to go take my vitamins."

Chapter Nineteen

WILL POWER

*I*t is a crisp fall morning, and Henry, having checked his yard, read his paper, and drunk his coffee, is ready to go downtown. He walks briskly down Freedom Street. *"Glad I wore my overcoat,"* he says to himself.

"Morning, Gus," he says as he rubs his hands against their coldness.

"Pumpkin time."

"Sure is. Got your Halloween face ready?"

"Keep it on all the time."

"Go on back. Looks like your buddies are all here."

Henry greets the group, and Joe says, "Your team messed up Saturday."

"Yes, if they'd just made that last field goal."

They continue their sports critique, as Violet takes their orders and returns to the kitchen.

"There's something wrong with Violet," says Victor. "She doesn't seem herself."

"Just a young girl on Monday morning. She'll be all right," pronounces Joe.

Henry draws his chair around and says, "As I told you last time, that was our last book. I've been over my notes. I think we have finished. You know all I can find out. Time for another project."

"Think we might take on perfecting the peace in the Middle East?" asks Roddy.

"Or poverty in America?"

"Or the dictators of China?"

"Why don't we just go back to generalized gossip?"

"I've got a serious project," says Will Mack. "This doesn't involve sitting around discussing interesting subjects--although I've enjoyed Henry's reports immensely, and am ready to sign up for another subject--it involves raising hell about the condition of so many nursing homes. You know what Vic told us about Fireball. It's outrageous that old people are treated with such disregard, are abused and exploited. I want them to start an investigation. Maybe we ought to do some investigation ourselves. I meant to bring some clippings and an article with me. I'll bring them next time."

"Maybe we ought to be more positive," says Rodney. "Even the best nursing homes need more personal attention by friends and people who want to be friends, because loneliness is so depressing. In addition to raising hell, we might start a regular visitors program. Take people for a walk, visit and talk, read to them if that is needed, and bring a little more brightness into their lives. You know we have some very good nursing homes, but even the best are dreary places. What can friends do?"

"I'm a volunteer right now," declares Victor. "Both ways. Let's get started."

"Sounds good to me," says Roddy, "and I want to thank Henry for doing such a great job. This has been terrific schooling for me. It's got me exercising, and I'm losing weight. Believe it or not, Henry, I am taking vitamins. You convinced me."

"Me, too," says Joe. "Henry, we've learned a lot. Chronic diseases, life expectancy, life span. . . ."

"And how the aging process probably works and . . . ."

"And how to cut down on the chances of stroke and heart attack and cancer. . . ."

"And organ reserve and how maybe to slow down aging and brace against the ills of old age," says Victor.

"And we know we might well go out swinging--with a little bit of luck."

"And not so soon!"

"And the Final Four--so simple to remember how to fight off age and illness and limping," says Roddy.

"Name them!" says Henry.

"Sure we can," both Joe and Victor speak at once.

"Eat right. Cut down on fats."

"And sugar. . . ."

"Get calcium, dodge salt. . . ."

"Eat balanced meals, and take carefully chosen vitamin supplements," says Rodney.

"Keep your weight down," says Lear. "Beer bellies breed strokes. Eat sparse."

"Second?"

"Hold down drinking and quit smoking," says Victor.

"Next?"

"Get physical exams."

"And examine yourselves."

"Fourth? Exercise! Don't quit," says Joe. "Exercise. Build muscle. Don't get lazy."

"Excellent," says Henry. "A's for all of you. And of course there are other things, more mental than physical. Keep involved. Care about others. Use your brain. Stay active. What I've gotten out of all this is that it can be exciting to fight old age. It is as exciting a challenge as we have ever had in our lives."

"Sure is--to beat the odds. That is what we have been trying to do in everything else since the first grade. Beat the odds."

"With luck," adds Joe.

"Knock it, Joe," says Roddy. "You know you make your own luck."

"That's what I meant," says Joe.

Violet comes back in with a plate of eggs and bacon in her right hand, which she puts in front of Lear, and a bowl of corn flakes in her left hand, which she moves back and forth under Will Mack's nose. At first he doesn't notice. He is talking to Joe.

Suddenly he looks and exclaims, "Violet, what is that sparkling thing on your finger!"

Before she can answer, everybody is involved.

"Violet, it is beautiful. Who gave it to you?"

"Who is the lucky fellow?"

Violet blushes, stammers, "Do you like it?"

"Love it. Who is he?"

Violet steps back, tucks her head. "John McCorn," she quietly says.

"John McCorn!" Will Mack screams. "That sneak. How did he do this without our knowing?"

"Wonderful, wonderful," says Henry. "I've been hoping this would happen."

"You knew?"

"Well, just hoped."

"Tell us about it, Violet."

"Nothing to tell. He gave it to me last night. Mama went on to bed like I told her she had to."

"Did he get down on his knee to propose," Roddy asks.

"I'm not going to tell you all that." Violet is blushing. "He did say to tell all of you that he wanted you to be his pallbearers."

"Pallbearers!"

"You know how Johnny is, always teasing. He wants you all to be in the wedding. It's going to be in the church. Mama is making my dress, already had it about half done. I want Mr. Murphy to give me away."

"Violet, I'd be honored," says Henry. "You'll make a beautiful bride."

"Thank you, Mr. Henry." Violet is crying.

"Well, now," says Roddy, "cut out that bawling, and let's get down to business. When is the great day?"

"December first."

"Great, we'll be there," says Zaroom.

"Now you'll be leaving us. I don't think I can stand it," says Victor.

"Not right away. We're going on a honeymoon. Then I'm going to work until we get enough to put a down payment on a house. Johnny is going to keep his job for about three months. Then he's going to start his own business."

By this time everybody is standing, including a half dozen other customers who have joined the party.

"Sit down, Violet," Joe commands. "I'm going to be the waiter. Don't order. I'm going to bring your breakfast."

"I've already eaten," Violet blushes.

"Never mind, I'm going to serve you. Gus, you got any champagne?" he yells at Gus who is about half way from the cash register, not quite knowing what to make of all this.

Gus brings out two bottles of Greek wine, and Joe pours it around in water tumblers.

"Here's to the beautiful bride," Lear lifts his glass.

"The bride, the bride!"

Violet picks anxiously at the heaping plate of eggs, potatoes, sausage, and toast that Joe has brought her, then stands up. "I've got to go to work."

She starts scurrying around to pick up the dishes but no one has eaten. Then she nervously pours hot coffee and retreats to the kitchen.

"Well sir," says Victor, "a great ending for our school year. A great graduation."

"Henry," says Roddy, "I don't know that I have ever enjoyed anything so much as your college of aging knowledge, to paraphrase Kay Kyser."

"Henry, you've been through all this, read ten times what you've sifted out for us. What is the most important thing for us to do?"

"All of it is important. We cut it down to four key moves."

"You can't dodge the question. One most important?"

"Fair enough. Exercise--muscle strength and physical condition. Three observations: Most all else depends on and is made easier by good physical condition. It is tempting to avoid exercise, to put it off, to quit. Because exercise is the toughest assignment you have given yourself, if you do this one as promised, you likely will do all the other things you have promised yourself.

"That's it."

"Henry, we can never thank you enough."

"It's been great. Thank you."

No one says anything much, as they more or less finish their breakfasts.

Lear finally speaks. "Gentlemen," he says, "this has been great. Henry, your lessons have been terrific."

Lear then takes a long draw on his cigarette, and slowly blows smoke rings across the table.

When the last one fades away, he says, "All that we need now is will power."

BIBLIOGRAPHY

My purpose was not to write a scientific treatise, but to draw out of the research and literature just so much as the average aging person would need to know. The works cited are to suggest additional readings for those who might want to pursue further some aspect of the subject, and also to list the literature on which I have relied as I wrote this presentation. I decided not to use footnotes. They seemed so out of place. I got ahold of Henry's little cards. Here they are.

Adelman, Richard C. and George S. Roth. *Testing the Theories of Aging*. Boca Raton, Florida: CRC Press, 1982.

An interesting and comprehensive account and evaluation by a number of scientists on various theories of aging, a fascinating subject. The genetic theories, pathology of aging, free radical theory, error theories, and cellular aging are subjects included, and a chapter on autoimmunity and aging by Susan Gottesman and Roy Walford, are areas covered. This book was published recently, in 1982, but there has been a rapid advance in research since then.

"Age Page." The National Institute of Aging of the Food and Drug Administration. Periodic issues.

"Anti-aging." *Consumer Reports*. January 1992.

Atchley, Robert C. *Aging, Continuity and Change.* Belmont, California: Wadsworth, 1983.

Bakerman, Seymour, ed. *Aging Life Processes.* Springfield, Illinois: Charles C. Thomas, Publisher, 1969.
    Very good basic background. Although over 20 years have passed since this book was written, I would consider it required reading for students of the subject.

Baltes, Paul B. and Margaret M. Baltes. *Successful Aging: Perspectives from the Behavioral Sciences.* New York: Cambridge University Press, 1990.
    This book originated with a workshop sponsored by the European Science Foundation, with some two dozen contributors, one-third from the United States, and the remainder from Europe. The first purpose was to explore the nature of successful aging, its conditions and its variations. Considers psychological perspectives, medical perspectives, cognitive functioning, memory, bereavement, coping, adjusting, and selfhood, among other subjects.

Bernstein, Carol. *Aging, Sex, and DNA Repair.* San Diego: Academic Press, 1992.
    "Aging as we will argue, is mainly the accumulation of unrepaired DNA damages in somatic cells." Our question is how to avoid and repair DNA damage.

Birren, James E., R. Bruce Sloane, and Gene D. Dohan, eds. *Handbook of Aging and the Individual: Psychological and Biological Aspects.* Chicago: University of Chicago Press, 1959.
    This book gave me a fundamental start in spite of its age.

------, **and Vern L. Bengtson, Eds.** *Emergent Theories of Aging.* New York: Springer Publishing Company, 1988.
    Excellent authoritative, comprehensive textbook by recognized leaders in the several fields discussed. It will not tell one as much about aging as about how science expects to find out

more. Valuable to understand direction of research on various theories.

Bogdonoff, Morton D. *Forever Fit: The Exercise Program for Staying Young.* Boston: Little, Brown, 1983.

A clear set of recommendations for an exercise program, workable and feasible for older people, drawn from the author's experience with the Duke Longitudinal Studies; a reference book well worth owning.

Bolin, Arthur. See Adelman and Roth.

Borz, Walter M. *We Live Too Short and Die Too Long.* New York: Bantam Books, 1991.

This is a readable, understandable, optimistic, even jolly, book written for general consumption. It is based on science as well as reason, if indeed they are not the same, and is well worth reading. Dr. Bortz practiced and researched with his father, Dr. Edward L. Bortz.

Brazil, Mary Jo. *Building Library Collections on Aging: A Selection Guide and Core List.* Santa Barbara, California: ABC-CLIO, 1990.

Useful for identifying library materials, books, periodicals, videos, etc.

Busse, Ewald W., George L. Maddox, and E. Edward Buckley. *The Duke Longitudinal Studies of Normal Aging, 1955-1980 Overview of History, Design, and Findings.* New York: Springer Publishing Company, 1985.

Dr. Busse is a distinguished pioneer in the studies of aging, having originated the Duke University Center for the study of Aging.

The book is included in the bibliography because of the importance of these studies to the understanding of aging, and as pioneer efforts in the longitudinal approach to research in this field, and because it further defines three publications that are a part of this bibliography.

Butler, Robert N., and Alex G. Bearn , eds. *The Aging Process: Therapeutic Implications.* New York: Raven Press, 1984.

This is a summary of the Merck Sharp & Dohme International Medical Advisory Council, and is dated, but it lays out the basics of a number of areas of interest, such as the biology of aging and genotropic theories, physiological changes, and various aspects of medication.

Chapman, Nancy. *Dietary Practices of Older People: Assessing the Benefits and Risks.* Washington, D.C.: N. Chapman Associates, Inc., February 1990.

This review of the use of supplements, as well as the nutrient needs, seems to be objective. It has the ring of truth.

Charness, Neil, Ed. *Aging and Human Performance.* New York: John Wiley & Sons, 1985.

This book contains nine articles covering "a wide variety of domains: sensory and perceptual, memory, spatial reasoning, problem-solving, physical performance, and workplace performance....The remaining thread running through the volume is...one of the more hopeful trends...for improving the performance of older people....You can 'train an old dog to do new tricks,' as has been shown numerous times in recent investigations."

Chernoff, Ronni. Ed. *Geriatric Nutrition: The Health Professional's Handbook.* Gaithersburg, Maryland: Aspen Publishers, Inc. 1991.

This book, as its title indicates, is for the health professional. It is written and arranged in a manner to be readily informative for the non-professional. Some twenty-three distinguished scientists have contributed the seventeen chapters.

Comfort, Alex. *A Good Age.* New York: Crown Publishers, Inc., 1976.

This is a book for all people looking with excitement to growing older.

------ *Ageing: The Biology of Senescence*. London: Routledge & Kegan Paul, 1956.

A classic. One of the early modern books, by one of the pioneers, reviewing the field and calling for more research and attention to the field.

------ *Say Yes to Old Age: Developing a Positive Attitude Toward Aging*. New York: Crown Publishers, Inc., 1990.

This is a book that should be read by all who are old and all who expect to be old. Written by one of the modern pioneer researchers in ageing (the British spelling in the title of an early work of his), it is uplifting and enlightening, and a pleasure to read.

Cooper, Edwin L. Ed. *Stress, Immunity, and Aging*. New York: M. Dekker, 1984.

While this book, a series of articles, contains information far beyond the knowledge needed by most laymen, it is an exciting display of the emerging understanding of the relationship between the body's defense system and stress, and the connection with aging.

Cornaro, Louis. *The Art of Living Long: The Temperate Life*. In William F. Butler, *Four Discourses*. Milwaukee, Wisconsin, 1903.

Cousins, Norman. *Anatomy of Illness*. New York: Norton, 1979.

This is the remarkable story of Cousins's remarkable recovery from a deadly disease.

------. *The Healing Heart: Antidotes to Panic and Helplessness*. New York: W.W. Norton & Company, Inc., 1983. Cousins is always worth reading.

------. *Head First: the Biology of Hope*. New York: Dutton, 1992

Crapo, Lawrence M., and James F. Fries. *Vitality and Aging*. San Francisco: W.H. Freeman and Company, 1981.

This book is a delightfully written overview of the subject. It is well worth reading--and keeping.

Curtis, Howard J. *Biological Mechanisms of Aging*. Springfield Illinois: Charles C. Thomas, Publisher, 1966.

Cutler, Richard G., *Cellular Aging: Concepts and Mechanisms*. New York: Published by Basil, 1976.

Diet and Health, Report of a study by the Committee on Diet and Health, in consultation with the Food and Nutrition Board, the Commission on Life Sciences, and the National Research Council. Washington, D.C.: National Academy Press, 1989.

Dil'man, V.M., M. Rosenberg, translator. *The Grand Biological Clock*. Moscow: Mir Publishers. Chicago: Imported by Imported Publications, 1989.

This is a clear discussion of the various theories of aging, more than needed for my purposes, but is well worth studying by those whose interests point them in this direction. Fascinating descriptions of cells, endocrine system, the pituitary gland and the hypothalamus, and all the rest.

There is an excellent discussion of the cancer process in Chapter 10, which is beyond the intended scope of my book. I will note several quotations: ". . . figuratively speaking, higher organisms burn away in the flame of fats during aging." He also notes that "aging is a disease of regulation and, therefore many aspects of it can be subjected to treatment." Free radicals, he points out, "can react with DNA and proteins which induce mutations and other damage."

Eisdorfer, Carl, and Cohen, Donna, *Mental Health Care of the Aging: A Multidisciplinary Curriculum for Professional Training*. New York: Springer Publishing Company.

Eisdorfer, Carl and Lawton, M. Powell, Editors, *The Psychology of Adult Development and Aging.* Washington, D.C.: American Psychological Association, 1973.

Evans, William and Irwin H. Rosenberg, with Jacqueline Thompson. *Biomarkers: The 10 Determinants of Aging You Can Control.* New York: Simon & Schuster, 1991.
    This is a good book for a non-specialist, full of useful advice, and worth having in one's library.

Fabris, Fabrizio, Luigi Pernigotti, and Ermanno Ferrario, Eds. *Sedentary Life and Nutrition.* New York: Raven Press, 1990.
    This is volume 38 in an "Aging Series" by this publisher. There are 47 contributors, all established scientists in universities and medical institutions, most Italian, with about a dozen from other European countries. The volume includes a series of interesting articles, including subjects of motor behavior and nutrition, and nutrition and various diseases, among others. The editors make three points in their preface: Sedentary life undermines both the biological and psychosocial integrity of the elderly subject. Mental habits may deeply affect the individual aging process and some age-related diseases. There are consistent possibilities for preventing some of the most severe disorders of the aging process.

Family Medical Guide. American Medical Association.
    A good reference book.

Family Medicine Guide. Consumer Guide.
    A good reference book.

Feltman, John and Editors of Prevention magazine Health Books. *Food and Nutrition.* Emmans, PA: Rodale press, Inc., 1993.

Finch, Caleb Elicott. *Longevity, Senescence, and the Genome.* Chicago: University of Chicago Press, 1990.

A very thorough textbook covering the biology of senescence and the genomic functions during senescence. Not for the general reader. A major theme is, "What role does the genome have in the mechanisms that may be pacemakers for senescence and lifespan?" A conclusion is that "many aspects of senescence should be strongly modifiable by interventions at the level of gene expression."

Fischer, Ed and Jane Thomas Noland. *What's So Funny About Getting Old?* Minneapolis, Minnesota: CompCare Publishers, 1991.

Jokes are also mostly getting old, but not a bad Father's Day present.

Foner, Anne. *Aging and Old Age: New Perspectives.* Englewood Cliffs, New Jersey: Prentice-Hall, Inc., 1986.

This book, published as a part of a modern sociology series, is a good definition of the position, plight, and promise of the aging person in society.

Fries, James F. *Aging Well.* Reading, Massachusetts: Addison-Wesley Publishing Company, 1989.

This is a book that should be kept at home as a reference. It is inclusive, authoritative, and well-organized. Of course it should be read before it is kept.

------. *Arthritis: A Comprehensive Guide.* Reading, Massachusetts: Addison-Wesley Publishing Company, 1990.

Frolkis, V.V. *Aging and Life-Prolonging Processes.* Translated from the Russian by Nicholas Bobrov. New York: Springer Verlag, 1982.

This is a Russian scientist who advanced the theory of "vitauct." It is fairly technical, but is a good discussion of aging and the glandular and chemical mechanisms of aging, the brain and aging, as well as life-prolongation experiments, and a general discussion of life span and aging.

------. *Life Span Prolongation.* Nailja G. Edelsburg, translator. Boca Raton: CRC Press, 1991.

A thorough study of aging and anti-aging processes, including the idea of vitauct.

Gilmore, Grover C., Peter J. Whitehouse, and May L. Wykkle, Eds., *Memory, Aging, and Dementia: Theory, Assessment, and Treatment.* New York: Springer Publishing Company, 1989.

This book grew out of the conference held in Cleveland, October 1987, sponsored by the University Center on Aging and Health of Case Western Reserve University and the Alzheimer Center of University Hospitals of Cleveland. It includes articles on the memory processes, impairment of memory and everyday memory problems of the aged, as well as considerable discussion of Alzheimer's disease.

Havel, Richard J., ed. *Recommended Dietary Allowances.* Washington, D.C.: National Academy Press, 1989.

Hayflick, Leonard. *How and Why We Age.* New York: Ballantine Books, c1994.

Hayflick, Leonard. In *The Geriatric Imperative.* Edited by Somers and Fabian. New York: Appelton-Century-Crofts, 1981.

Heart Attacks. U.S. Department of Health and Human Services. Washington, D.C.: U.S. Government Printing Office, 1986.

This booklet was adopted from a lecture delivered by Robert I. Levy when he was Director of the National Heart, Lung and Blood Institute. It is concise and well worth reading. The most recent updates can be obtained by writing: The National Heart, Lung and Blood Institute, The National Institutes of Health, 9000 Rockville Pike, Building 31, Room 4A21, Bethesda, Maryland 20892.

Hendler, Sheldon Saul. *The Complete Guide to Anti-Aging Nutrients.* New York: Simon and Schuster, 1985.

This is a very good discussion of anti-aging nutrients, the relationship of nutrition to aging, and suggested regimens.

Holeckova, Emma and Vincent J. Cristofalo. *Aging in Cell and Tissue Culture.* New York: Plenum Press, 1970.

Hypertension in Diabetes. U.S. Department of Health and Human Services. Bethesda, Maryland: Public Health Service, National Institutes of Health, 1985.

Johnson, John E., Jr., Denham Harman, Roy Walford, and Jaime Miquel, Eds. *Free Radicals, Aging, and Degenerative Diseases.* New York: Alan R. Liss, Inc., 1986.

This is a series of provocative articles by an impressive array of contributors, dealing with free radical theory of aging, the free radical process, the free radical relationship to various diseases, and protection against free radical damage.

Johnston, Priscilla W., ed. *Perspectives on Aging.* Cambridge, Massachusetts: Ballinger Publishing Company, 1981.

Katahn, Martin. *The T-Factor Diet.* New York: Bantam Books, 1989.

Lambert, Richard D., ed. *The Annals of the American Academy of Political and Social Science.* Vol. 503, May 1989.

Lansing, Albert I. "General Biology of Senescence." In James E. Birren, ed. *Handbook of Aging and the Individual.* Chicago: University of Chicago Press, 1959.

Lewis, Steven J. *Aging & Health: Linking Research and Public Policy.* Chelsea, Michigan: Lewis Publishers, Inc., 1989.

This is a report of a 1988 Saskatoon, Saskatchewan seminar on aging and health. Any book is worth perusing if its preface includes such comments as, "We considered it insufficiently challenging to hold the conference in a major city in a hospitable climate," and "We chose February in the hope that the expectation of bracing weather would weed out the triflers,..." and "The weather was, all things considered, perfect: --32C...."

I found useful to my understanding the sections related to medications, and research and a paper of Death, Ethics, and Choice, by Andrew Malcolm, and good section on financing of long-term care. I will admit to not having read the paper entitled, "Hip Fracture Trends in Saskatchawan, 1972-1984."

Lifelong Learning for an Aging Society. Special Committee on Aging, United States Senate. Washington, D.C.: U.S. Government Printing Office, 1991.

Lindbergh, Anne Morrow. *Gift from the Sea*. New York: Pantheon Books, 1955; 1975.
A wonderful little classic.

Lonergan, Edmund T. Ed. *Extending Life, Enhancing Life: A National Research Agenda on Aging*. Washington, D.C.: National Academy Press, 1991.

Ludwig, Frederic C. *Life Span Extension--Consequences and Open Questions*. New York: Springer Publishing Company, 1991.

Maddox, George L., Ed.-in-Chief. *The Encyclopedia of Aging*. New York: Springer Publishing company, 1987.
A magnificent and comprehensive encyclopedia, with six editors and 224 contributors. New Edition, 1995.

Maddox, George L., Editor. *The Future of Aging and the Aged*. Atlanta, Georgia: Southern Newspaper Publishers Assoc. Fdn., 1971.

Man and His Years, Health Publications Inc., Raleigh, North Carolina, 1951.
This is an account of the first National Conference on Aging, sponsored by the Federal Security Agency. President Harry Truman wrote an introduction, a letter to Oscar R. Ewing, the

Federal Security Administrator. Mr. Truman wrote, "I should like therefore to ask you to explore... the problems incident to our increasingly older population...." He had defined the scope: "While problems of income and maintenance are of great importance to them [older persons], other aspects of life, such as their participation as citizens in our democracy, their housing, recreation, education, physical and mental health, are significant."

The first chapter is Oscar Ewing's statement to the Conference. Jack Ewing was one of the giants of public service of that era. Later, in retirement, and living in Chapel Hill, he was of crucial help in getting established in North Carolina's Research Triangle Park the laboratories of the National Institute of Environmental Health, of the National Institutes of Health.

He wrote: "What shall we do about our old people? Shall we ignore them and dissipate the most mature years of their lives, so that they become meaningless as people and as part of our national community? Or shall we look upon their experience, skills, wisdom and judgment as great national assets which, if properly realized, could serve the country well while giving added meaning to their added years? Having made life longer, we must now work to make longer life worthwhile."

This book provides a workable base line. Now some 40 years since its formulation, the deliberations of 816 participants of subjects from income and employment, to health, education and recreation, to family life, to research and projected action, set forth the dimensions of aging in what has now become a lasting historical reference.

Morley, John E., Zvi Glick, Laurence Z. Rubenstein, Eds. *Geriatric Nutrition: A Comprehensive Review.* New York: Raven Press, 1990.

Rather technical discussion of diet and nutrients in relation to diabetes, hypertension, cardiovascular and other diseases.

Moser, Marvin. *High Blood Pressure: What You can do About it.* Elmsford, New York: The Benjamin Company, Inc., 1977; 1987.

Good, but essentially beyond the scope of this discussion.

Nagatsu, Toshiharu and Osamu, Hayaishi. Eds. *Aging of the Brain: Cellular and Molecular Aspects of Brain Aging and Alzheimer's Disease.* Basel, New York: Karger, 1990.

This is an authoritative book in highly technical style, a series of reports at a symposium of scientists, and is not easily utilized by the non-scientist. There is a general, and obvious, conclusion, namely that there remains much unknown in the realm of the aging brain, and a general confidence that the increased interest and the new genetic techniques (e.g. DNA, gene grafting) in science hold much promise for future discourse in the cause, prevention, and treatment of Parkinson's, Alzheimer's and other disorders of the brain.

1971 White House Conference on Aging, U.S. government Printing Office, Washington, D.C., 1971.

This document is a Senate print of the report of the Conference, and might be read in conjunction with *Man and His Years,* and reflects more of a legislative look at aging, and is a product of the Senate Special Committee on Aging.

Normal Human Aging: The Baltimore Longitudinal Study of Aging. National Institutes of Health, Publication 84-2450, 1984.

Nutrition: A Lifelong Concern. U.S. Department of Health and Human Services. September 1984.

Ory, Marcia G. and Kathleen Bond. *Aging and Health Care: Social Science Perspectives.* New York: Routledge, ?

Palmore, Erdman, ed. *Normal Aging II: Reports from the Duke Longitudinal Studies, 1970-1973.* Durham, North Carolina: Duke University Press, 1974.

A landmark sequence to a landmark study.

------ **and Ewald W. Busse.** *Normal Aging III: Reports from the Duke Longitudinal Studies, 1975-1984.* Durham, North Carolina: Duke University Press, 1985.

Fundamental and essential information on physical, psychological, and social aging, mental health and mental illness, with contributions by dozens of distinguished scholars. A sequel to Normal Aging II, and Social Patterns in Normal Aging. The Duke Longitudinal studies originated are landmarks in the field of gerontology.

------. *Social Patterns in Normal Aging: Findings from the Duke Longitudinal Studies.* Durham: Duke University Press, 1981.

This book notes the end of the two decades at the Duke Center for the Study of Aging and Human Development of the Duke Longitudinal Studies, under the leadership of Ewald W. Busse, M.D. The "Studies documented effectively a realistically optimistic view of adult life in all its variety. Older adults demonstrably have far greater biological, psychological, and social potential than had been imagined previously." The foreward, from which this quotation comes, was written by George L. Maddox, Ph.D., who followed Dr. Busse as director of the Center.

Pauling, Linus. *How to Live Longer and Feel Better.* New York: W.H. Freeman, 1986.

Perlmutter, Marion, Ed. *Late Life Potential.* Washington, D.C.: Gerontological Society of America, 1990.

A symposium of the Gerontological Society of America, relating aging to the subjects of physical performance, cognitive capacity, mental abilities, wisdom and creativity.

Poon, Leonard W., James L. Fozard, Laird S. Cermak, David Arenberg, and Larry W. Thompson, eds. *New Directions in Memory and Aging: Proceedings of the George A. Talland Memorial Conference, Boston 1978.* Hillsdale, New Jersey: Lawrence Erlbaum Associates, Publishers, 1980.

Quackery, a $10 Billion Scandal. Washington, D.C.: House of Representatives, Ninety-Eighth Congress, Second session, 1984.

Report of the Expert Panel on Detection, Evaluation, and Treatment of High Blood Cholesterol in Adults. U.S. Department of Health and Human Services, 1989.

Research on Aging Act, 1973. Washington, D.C.: U.S. Government Printing Office, 1974.

Riley, Matilda White and John W. Riley, Jr. eds. "The Quality of Aging: Strategies for Intervention." In *The Annals of the American Academy of Political and Social Science,* Richard D. Lambert, ed.

Rogers, Spencer L. *The Aging Skeleton.* Springfield, Illinois: Charles C. Thomas, 1982.
    Very fine treatise on bones and bone disorders in advanced age.

Rosenthal, Evelyn R., Ed. *Women, Aging, and Ageism.* New York: Haworth Press, 1990.
    Case studies and other writings about women, poignant situations, isolation and ostracization, bound to an individual, angry at life, caught in hopeless care-giving situations for years on end. The lessons? Don't abandon friends who are caught in this kind of pain and isolation. Don't overlook neighbors. It is most often much tougher on women than on men who suffer such situations. Women frequently have less chance than men to overcome the loneliness of old age.

Simpson, Ida Harper, and McKinney, John C., eds. *Social Aspects of Aging.* Durham, North Carolina: Duke University Press, 1966.

Somers, Anne R. and Dorothy R. Fabian. *The Geriatric Imperative: An Introduction to Gerontology and Clinical Geriatrics.* New York: Appleton-Century-Crofts, 1981.
    This is a wide-ranging, readable, and extremely useful survey of the field, including articles on patient care, education in geriatrics, national policy, and research in numerous aspects of aging. The editors, both of the College of Medicine and Den-

tistry of New Jersey-Rutgers Medical School, tell us that the book and most of the chapters grew out of a Faculty Research Seminar on Geriatrics and Gerontology sponsored by their College.

Stroke Update. U.S. Department of Health and Human Services. Bethesda, Maryland: Office of Clinical Center Communications, National Institutes of Health, 1988.

A concise summary. Later editions can be obtained by writing: The National Institutes of Neurological and Communicative Disorders and Stroke, National Institutes of Health, 9000 Rockville Pike, Building 31, Room 8AD6, Bethesda, Maryland 20892.

So You Have High Blood Cholesterol. U.S. Department of Health and Human Services, 1989.

Spirduso, Waneen W. and Helen M. Eckert, Eds. *Physical Activity and Aging.* American Academy of Physical Education Papers, No. 22. Champaign, Illinois: Human Kinetics Books, 1989.

Authorities in physical activity address contributions of health, fitness, and motor skills to successful aging. The topics include psychomotor changes, skeletal muscle weakness, physical activity relative to hypertension, cardiovascular function and the central nervous system, and exercise prescriptions, among other subjects. Bonnie G. Berger on physical activity and life quality is very good.

Staudinger, Ursula M., Steven.W. Cornelius, and Paul B. Baltes. "The Aging of Intelligence: Potential and Limits." *The Annals of The American Academy of Political and Social Science.* Eds. Richard D. Lambert and Alan W. Heston. London: Sage Publications, 1989.

The Relationship Between Nutrition, Aging, and Health: A Personal and Social Challenge. Hearing Before the Special Committee on Aging, United States Senate, Ninety-ninth Congress, First Session, Albu-

querque, *New Mexico, December 14, 1985.* Washington, D.C.: Government Printing Office, 1986.

The Surgeon General's Report on Nutrition and Health. U.S. Department of Health and Human Services, Public Health Service. Washington, D.C.: U.S. Government Printing Office, 1988.

Prepared under the auspices of the Nutrition Policy Board, U.S. Department of Health and Human Services, which includes six medical doctors and four other officers in administrative positions with the Public Health Service and Advisors, working group members, drafters, and reviewers numbering more than 200, this Report is understandably vague and tentative in places. The section on Aging and Nutrition takes 22 pages of 712, and is worth reading, and certainly that remainder of the Report is a valuable reference book.

Torach, Richard M. *The Brain is Younger Than You Think.* Chicago: Nelson-Hall, 1981.

Good discussions of the relationship of aging with memory loss, acute confusion, depression, the brain condition, senility, and mental illness.

Vickery, Donald and James Fries. *Take Care of Yourself.* Reading, Massachusetts: Addison-Wesley Publishing Company, 1989.

Vierck, Elizabeth. *Fact Book on Aging.* Santa Barbara, California: ABC-CLIO, 1990.

"One-liners," as described in the preface, tell us statistically how many seniors living alone rent, how many have elevated blood pressure, and how many are trying to lose weight. Good stuff, if you need to know so many facts. The statistics are, we are told, "representative of every eighth American." Okay.

Walford, Roy L. *Maximum Life Span.* New York: W.W. Norton, 1983.

Very interesting for rats. Can it be applied to humans? It certainly has some lessons and promise for humans.

Warner, Huber R., Ed. *Modern Biological Theories of Aging.* New York: Raven Press, 1987.

Watt, Bernice K. and Annabel L. Merrill. *Composition of Foods.* Washington, D.C.: U.S. Government Printing Office, 1975.

Weindruch, Richard and Roy L. Walford. The *Retardation of Aging and Disease by Dietary Restriction.* Springfield, Illinois: Charles C Thomas, Publisher, 1988.

This fascinating and readable book follows Walford's *Maximum Life Span*, about a revolutionary, if not recent, concept that dietary restriction might retard aging in human beings. There is no evidence that this regimen can be successful for people who are already at the age considered elderly. There is argument that dietary restriction is beneficial, in any event.

Williams, T. Franklin. *Rehabilitation in the Aging.* New York: Raven Press, 1984.